Boost Your
BREAST MILK

AN ALL-IN-ONE GUIDE FOR NURSING MOTHERS TO BUILD A HEALTHY MILK SUPPLY

ALICIA C. SIMPSON MS, RD, IBCLC, LD

THE EXPERIMENT

NEW YORK

Boost Your Breast Milk: *An All-in-One Guide for Nursing Mothers to Build a Healthy Milk Supply*

Copyright © 2017 by Alicia C. Simpson

The Experiment, LLC, 220 East 23rd Street, Suite 301, New York, NY 10010-4674
theexperimentpublishing.com

Neither the author nor the publisher is engaged in rendering professional advice or services to individual readers and their children or relatives. The ideas, procedures, and suggestions in this book are not intended as a substitute for consulting a physician. All matters regarding health require medical supervision. Neither the author nor the publisher shall be liable or responsible for any loss, injury, or damage allegedly arising from any information or suggestion in this book. The opinions expressed in this book represent the personal views of the author and not of the publisher.

Many of the designations used by manufacturers and sellers to distinguish their products are claimed as trademarks. Where those designations appear in this book and The Experiment was aware of a trademark claim, the designations have been capitalized.

The Experiment's books are available at special discounts when purchased in bulk for premiums and sales promotions as well as for fund-raising or educational use. For details, contact us at info@ theexperimentpublishing.com.

Library of Congress Cataloging-in-Publication

Names: Simpson, Alicia C., author.
Title: Boost your breast milk : an all-in-one guide for nursing mothers to
  build a healthy milk supply / Alicia C. Simpson MS, RD, IBCLC, LD.
Description: New York : The Experiment, [2017]
Identifiers: LCCN 2016020921 (print) | LCCN 2016029908 (ebook) | ISBN
  9781615193462 (pbk.) | ISBN 9781615193479 (ebook)
Subjects: LCSH: Breastfeeding. | Breastfeeding--Health aspects. |
  Lactation--Nutritional aspects.
Classification: LCC RJ216 .S4628 2017 (print) | LCC RJ216 (ebook) | DDC
  613.2/69--dc23
LC record available at https://lccn.loc.gov/2016020921

ISBN 978-1-61519-346-2
Ebook ISBN 978-1-61519-347-9

Cover design by Sarah Schneider | Text design by Pauline Neuwirth
Cover and interior illustrations by Kondrateva Ekaterina
Author photograph by Kelly Donovan

Manufactured in the United States of America
Distributed by Workman Publishing Company, Inc.
Distributed simultaneously in Canada by Thomas Allen & Son Ltd.

First printing February 2017
10 9 8 7 6 5 4 3 2 1

*To my life's greatest teacher and my
endless source of joy—my Bradley.
Hello my love.*

CONTENTS

Introduction   xi

PART I

Breastfeeding 101

1 WHAT YOU NEED TO KNOW TO START NURSING   2

Preparing to Nurse   3

Building and Maintaining a Healthy Supply   4

2 THE BASICS OF BREASTFEEDING   9

Latching   9

Positioning   11

Switching Breasts   16

Engorgement   17

Do I Need Breastfeeding Accessories?   18

Support   23

3 THE SCIENCE BEHIND MAKING MILK   25

The Stages of Milk Production   26

Milk-Making Hormones   28

PART II

The Myth of Low Milk Supply: Separating Fact from Fiction

4 AM I EXPERIENCING LOW MILK SUPPLY OR TRANSFER?   32

Evaluating Your Milk Supply   33

Is My Baby Getting Enough Milk?   35

5 MEDICAL REASONS FOR LOW MILK SUPPLY   39

Breast Reduction Surgery   39

Mastitis and Plugged Ducts   40

Insufficient Glandular Tissue   42

Polycystic Ovary Syndrome (PCOS)   43

Thyroid Issues   44

Prolactin Deficiency   46

Infertility Secondary to Pituitary Disorders   47

Sheehan's Syndrome   47

Hormonal Birth Control   48

Infant Anatomical Abnormalities   50

Birthing Methods and Medications Given During Birth   54

Retained Placenta   55

Preterm Births   55

Overweight and Obesity   56

6 NONMEDICAL REASONS FOR LOW MILK SUPPLY   58

Ineffective Suck or Latch   59

Nipple Shields   61

Supplementing with Formula   63

Reducing or Eliminating Nighttime Feedings   68

Scheduling Feedings   70

Pacifier Use Between Feedings   71

Ineffective Milk Expression 72

Early Introduction of Solid Food 76

7 MILK SLUMPS **79**

Growth Spurts 79

Returning to Work or School 81

Welcome Back, Aunt Flo! 84

Stress 85

Malnutrition 85

PART III

Breastfeeding and Nutrition

8 NOURISHING YOUR BODY **90**

Managing Food Allergies and Breastfeeding 91

Maternal Energy Needs During Pregnancy and Lactation 91

Losing Weight While Breastfeeding 93

Macronutrient Needs of the Breastfeeding Woman 95

Micronutrient Needs of the Breastfeeding Woman 99

**9 BOOSTING YOUR BREAST MILK
THROUGH FOODS AND HERBS** **104**

Lactogenic Foods 105

Potential Lactogenic Foods and Herbs 113

Superfoods to Help You Breastfeed 114

Antilactogenic Foods, Herbs, and Medications 119

Other Foods to Avoid 122

10 FREQUENTLY ASKED QUESTIONS **125**

Are there any medications that have been
shown to improve milk supply? 125

Should I continue to take vitamins and supplements? 126

Can diet cause a fussy baby?   127

How do I know if my baby has a food allergy?   127

Can my diet affect the nutrient content
  or quality of my milk?   129

How do I choose the lactogenic foods
  that are right for me?   130

Are lactogenic foods and galactagogues
  safe for my family to eat?   130

Is it OK to take more than one galactagogue at a time?   131

How much water should I be drinking?   132

PART IV

The Recipes

A Note About the Recipes   134

Milk-Makin' Milks   136

Teas, Tonics, and Smoothies   144

Breakfast   150

Breads and Rolls   164

Side Dishes   170

Soups, Stews, and Salads   177

Dips, Bars, and Snacks   189

Entrées   196

Desserts   211

Notes   222

Acknowledgments   234

Index   236

About the Author   244

INTRODUCTION

When I am at the playground pushing my daughter on a swing and someone asks me what I do, I always reply with the simplest answer—I'm a dietitian and a lactation consultant. Without fail, each time, the person will open up to me about their breastfeeding journey or that of their partner, daughter, or other loved one. More often than not it's filled with more downs than ups and ultimately ends in early weaning. Mothers, fathers, grandparents, aunts, and uncles all share with me the struggles they've witnessed or experienced and how they wished they'd known where to look for help. Each time I hear these stories, my heart fills with a bit of pain because usually, breastfeeding issues are due to very fixable problems. Many times breastfeeding wasn't successful due to the wrong advice from the wrong person. When the mother needed support the most, there was no real support system in place to make her breastfeeding journey successful or even possible. This book seeks to change that.

On the simplest level, breast milk is food. And food is more complex than the sensory experience we have when we eat it or the nutrients we receive from it. It is essential to every component of our lives. Food dictates our physical, social, and mental health; it evokes strong emotional ties to our family, friends, culture, and subculture. Without it, life ceases to exist. The words *lactation* and *breastfeeding* are triggers for many people, and so, without even realizing it, most people breeze past the fact that I'm also a dietitian. I believe that breast milk elicits such a deep response from so many because it's the only food that a human makes organically. It's part of what defines us as mammals and links us to every other animal on the planet who nurses her young. Breast milk is the very first food that a human ever tastes, our very first experience with food. The act of breastfeeding teaches our bodies how to move, grow, and thrive. It builds bonds and strengthens us. It prepares us for life.

Breastfeeding is the biological norm for infant feeding. However, many people believe that, because breastfeeding is a normal and natural extension of pregnancy and the experience of having an infant, everything will just flow perfectly. When it doesn't, they might not know where to turn. For most mothers, all around the world and since the beginning of humankind, nursing has followed a predictable, easy pattern. For the majority of human existence, nearly all members of a society were nursed and witnessed nursing their whole lives. Challenges that arose with breastfeeding were typically quickly overcome because of the wisdom of the greater society. There was always a mother, grandmother, or friend who knew the answer. Breastfeeding was as much of a life skill passed down from generation to generation as any other form of hunting, gathering, or finding nourishment. Our world has since changed. Now, in Western societies, whole generations of families have gone without breastfeeding, and many people have never seen a child

nursing. The collective wisdom of communities has been replaced with misinformation and well-meaning, yet often incorrect, advice.

I myself can't recall a time in my childhood when I ever saw a woman nurse her child—although I can recall an infinite number of times I saw a child being bottle-fed formula. My daughter was the first child in over four generations of my family to be exclusively breastfed, but it wasn't easy. At the time she was born, I was finishing up my master's thesis on the sociocultural barriers to breastfeeding in the African American community and was preparing to sit for my dietetic certification as well as my board examination to become an International Board Certified Lactation Consultant. I had all the resources I needed and more to nurse my daughter, but it still wasn't without its moments of great difficulty. At first, I found myself struggling with sore, cracked, bleeding nipples. During the first year of my nursing journey, I had oversupply and severe engorgement, which made it difficult to breathe lying down and to consistently maintain a good latch. Then I went from having an oversupply that had allowed me to not only nurse my daughter but provide more than two thousand ounces of milk for donation, to a low supply almost overnight.

Looking back, my nursing experience provided me with the best education I could have ever received in supporting nursing mothers through their journeys. Although I was able to exclusively breastfeed without the use of formula or other supplements for more than four years, I was shocked that even with all the tools to help fix my nursing problems myself, I still battled many of the breastfeeding barriers that I had counseled so many women through. Ultimately, my battles and those of the women I've counseled led me right here to these pages, writing a book on breastfeeding, nutrition, and boosting your milk supply naturally through foods and herbs.

What can you expect to find inside? First, I'll cover the breastfeeding basics, including what you need to know about nursing, latching and positioning, and the science behind making milk. Then, in one of the most important parts of the book, The Myth of Low Milk Supply, I will give you all of the facts on evaluating your supply and why women experience milk slumps or low supply. Finally, after sharing what you need to know about nutrition during nursing, I'll provide you with a comprehensive list of nutrient-dense breastfeeding superfoods and lactogenic (milk-producing) foods— along with seventy-five original recipes that feature these amazing milk-makers and nutrient boosters. My hope is to share not only these delicious dishes and the science behind them, but the collective wisdom of generations of women who have breastfed all around the world. If you don't have a village of breastfeeding mothers around you or you're feeling lost in the endless sea of information that our modern world provides, this is your opportunity to learn, grow, and empower yourself!

PART ONE

Breastfeeding 101

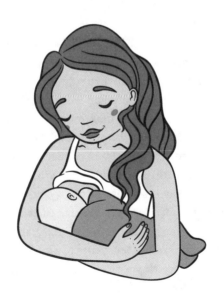

WHAT YOU NEED TO KNOW TO START NURSING

Pregnancy is a time of preparation. The first item on your to-do list is probably to prepare the nursery or rearrange your living space to accommodate your arriving little one. You make sure you have the requisite number of blankets, onesies, and burp cloths; research the right type of baby toys that will stimulate curiosity and learning in your newborn; and collect a stack of baby books by your bedside table that might take you until you have your next child to finish. You carefully go over your birth plan with your partner, listing all your expectations for how you would like to labor and deliver under the best of circumstances and making a list of backups for all those "just-in-case" moments. But even with the hours, days, and weeks of taking classes, reading books, and preparing for childbirth, something very important is usually missing—breastfeeding education. Which is odd, because even though I can confidently say that childbirth is a soul-changing experience (not only for yourself, but also for your partner and certainly for your new little one—who has just been pushed or pulled into the real world, ready or not!), labor and delivery last only a few hours to a few days. In contrast, your breastfeeding relationship with your child is one that has the potential to last for years. Yet, most of us aren't nearly as educated about breastfeeding as we think we are.

If you're currently balancing this book on top of a not-so-little bump that occasionally kicks your ribs and assaults your major organs with jabs and head-butts, then bravo to you! I applaud you for starting your journey to knowledge as soon as possible. If your baby has already arrived and you're in crisis mode frantically thumbing through the table of contents to find the section you need right now, then bravo to you, too! You're seeking out the information you need to empower yourself to make the best decisions for your family and to understand your body and your baby better.

PREPARING TO NURSE

No matter where you are in your journey, there are three things that I recommend as essential for every mom to do while pregnant and/or immediately postpartum to prepare to nurse:

1. Educate yourself. Many moms want to breastfeed but feel like the tools are just outside of their reach. Since you've picked up *Boost Your Breast Milk*, you have tool #1. The ultimate backup is *The Womanly Art of Breastfeeding* by Diane Wiessinger, Diana West, and Teresa Pitman. If you get any other book about breastfeeding, make it this one—even if you pick it up at your local library. The first time I picked it up, my daughter was already three months old and we had both willed ourselves through the first twelve weeks of breastfeeding. I had no time to actually sit down and read a book, so I finally dragged myself kicking and screaming into the twenty-first century and bought the book on Kindle. I flipped straight to the sections I was worried about— pain and sleep. The knowledge I was looking for not only helped me address those issues, it took away some of the fear I was feeling.

2. Take a breastfeeding class. All breastfeeding classes aren't made equal, but at the very least they'll teach you the basic mechanics of how to position your baby, what to expect, and most importantly what is and what is not normal. I lay out most of this information for you here, but repetition is important to remember and grasp skills. I highly recommend finding an International Board Certified Lactation Consultant (IBCLC) in your area and signing up for a breastfeeding class. If you're short on time or you can't find a class that's compatible with your schedule, try an online breastfeeding course. My company, Pea Pod Nutrition and Lactation Support, offers a variety of online classes, which you can find at peapodnutrition.org/classes/online.

3. Build your mommy tribe.
We all need each other. Nursing mothers from every species huddle close by each other—sharing information and learning from each other's triumphs and mistakes. Don't be afraid to form your own mommy tribe! It can be made up of any women you rely on or relate to. My own mommy tribe came from the most diverse, yet perfect, places. I met quite a few moms in my prenatal fitness and yoga classes, and I even met moms the first time I was sent to the hospital with a preterm labor scare. I've met moms at birthday parties, playing at the park, and walking through the botanical gardens. The beautiful tribe of moms I've befriended and fallen in love with help me through the daily struggles of motherhood and breastfeeding. Even when all was going well with nursing, it was still nice to have someone to call (or text) in the middle of the night who I could chat with about the fact that I had just soaked through my breast pads, pajama top, and bed, and now the baby was covered in breast milk. Only another mom could see that situation, tell me it was normal,

and give me great advice on how to move through it.

If you're already nursing (and are reading this book through the glare of your smartphone while silently praying your little one stays asleep for three more minutes so you can scroll to the chapter you need), don't worry—you haven't missed the boat. My list applies to all mothers in every stage of their breastfeeding journey. Having multiple resources to go to will help whether you need more information on breastfeeding, pumping, returning to work, sleeping, or introducing solids, and you will always need a mommy tribe. That will never change.

BUILDING AND MAINTAINING A HEALTHY SUPPLY

Moms want to know: What is the key to building a healthy milk supply? Is it pumping after each nursing session, taking fenugreek every day, or is it just a matter of luck? For a majority of women, building a healthy milk supply is as easy as breastfeeding when baby is hungry, avoiding bottles and artificial nipples until breastfeeding is well established, and allowing baby to suck for both nutritive and nonnutritive reasons.

The first key to maintaining a healthy milk supply is to breastfeed on demand. Don't watch the clock. Don't worry about how long your little one has been nursing or how long it has been between nursing sessions—just watch your baby. Find a comfortable nursing position, enlist all the support and help you need with the rest of life's to-do list, and take this time to feed your infant as much as she needs. You won't spoil your baby by nursing her too much, and you are not a pacifier—you are a mother. That means that every single time your child is at the breast, whether it's for food or for comfort, your baby is telling your body to make more milk. Once nursing is well established, you may want to read a good book, binge watch episodes of your favorite television shows, or listen to audiobooks and podcasts while nursing. All these things can help you move your focus away from watching the clock and instead allow you to relax into nursing.

The second key is to avoid introducing bottles, artificial nipples, or pacifiers until breastfeeding is well established. Suckling at the breast is a complex dance between sucking, swallowing, and breathing. Most newborns have a 10:1 suckswallow ratio, meaning that they will tend to suck ten times before taking a break to swallow and breathe. Infants learn by doing—the more an infant nurses, the stronger she gets and the more effective she becomes at not only nursing at the breast but balancing the dance of sucking, swallowing, and breathing. By approximately six to eight weeks of age, most full-term infants will have a 1:1 suck-swallow ratio, meaning they can suck, swallow, and breathe over and over again without tiring. While all forms of drinking require a certain degree of ability to balance these skills, bottle-feeding doesn't require that an infant actively suck. It doesn't promote the strengthening of the muscles in the jaw, head, and neck to facilitate a robust and active suck. Rather, bottle-feeding is a passive form of feeding: Breastfeeding is an active act that a baby must do, but bottle-feeding is an act of feeding done to the baby.

As long as a baby can swallow and breathe, she can typically bottle-feed. The ability to suck isn't needed.

Infants are just like us in many ways (after all, they're just tiny humans), and they'll seek out the easiest ways to get their needs met. Humans have invented an infinite number of ways to make our lives easier—from telephones, cars, and planes to the Internet and computers. To a newborn baby still learning how to suck, bottles are the ultimate in easy food delivery. They require little to no effort and provide enough nutrients to meet their needs. In fact, many babies fed with a bottle are overfed due to the passive method in which milk is transferred (see page 83 on how to make sure your baby isn't being overfed in the instances where she must be bottle-fed).

Some babies can easily go between suckling at the breast and passively drinking from a bottle with no problem. However, many babies find the task of nursing very difficult if they were fed with a bottle before they got a chance to properly learn to feed at the breast. Therefore, to help build a healthy milk supply and get nursing off to a great start, breastfeeding should be well established before a bottle is introduced. *Well established* means that your baby is transferring milk well, gaining weight appropriately, and has an appropriate wet- and poopy-diaper count for her age, and both mother and baby feel comfort and no pain while nursing.

There are dozens of reasons that an infant might be supplemented in the first weeks of life: Sometimes infants have a medical need that requires the use of additional feedings beyond the breast, or mother has an unexpected separation from her baby before breastfeeding is well established, such as in cases where infants are in the NICU or mother and baby aren't discharged from the hospital at the same time. If any of these scenarios happens to you, ask your hospital or lactation consultant to provide you with an alternative method of feeding. While bottles are the easiest way to supplement, they are certainly not the only way. Infants can be finger-fed with a supplemental nursing system (SNS), which uses a tube taped to the finger and connected to a bottle; through a needle-less syringe; by cup; by spoon; or by a variety of other easy-to-make-or-find feeding systems designed specifically to help ensure that infants don't form an aversion to the breast and a preference for the bottle.

The third key to building and maintaining a healthy supply is to nurse your little one whether it's for nutritive or nonnutritive reasons. Many mothers not only fear that their little one will "use them as a pacifier" but are actively warned about doing so from well-meaning friends and loved ones. However, this misguided advice doesn't take into account the natural need for an infant to suck at the breast for both nutritive and nonnutritive purposes. No matter what anyone tells you, you are not a pacifier; you are a mother. You are not a piece of plastic or mass-produced silicone; you are the source of the heartbeat your child has used as a soundtrack to her entire life thus far. You are your child's only source of nourishment, the most familiar source of comfort, and the only home that she knows. This new world your little one has been thrust into is a scary one! Her previous world was wet, dark, and relatively quiet. In contrast, this world is dry, bright, and incredibly noisy. Sensory life in utero and in the real world are polar-opposite experiences. For this reason and so many others, your little one will turn to you first when she needs comfort, and nursing provides the ultimate comfort at this time in her life, often completely eliminating the need for a pacifier in the early weeks postpartum.

All sucking, whether nutritive or nonnutritive, stimulates your breast to make more milk. Every time your infant suckles at the breast, she's telling your body to make more. No suck is a wasted suck. During times when nursing is taking a bit longer than usual and your infant appears to have changed from an active to a nonnutritive suck, simply try nursing in the side-lying position (page 16) where you can both lie down and relax. Instead of watching the clock, use the distraction techniques I discussed earlier in this section—catch up on your favorite show, read a book, or check in with your friends on social media. You'll be surprised how good you get at multitasking the longer you nurse.

Your baby will become more independent and more self-assured as time goes on. Every day, with your loving guidance, your child will come one step closer to finding her way in the world. For this very short period in time, your baby needs you more than anything else. These three keys—breastfeeding on demand, not using a bottle or other articifical nipples until breastfeeding is well established, and remembering to allow nonnutrive sucking to help stimulate milk production—will help ensure that you have enough milk to meet your infant's nutrient needs and have a long, successful breastfeeding relationship. It seems so simple, but American culture is usually one in which infant independence is praised and infant attachment chastised. It can be overwhelming for a new mom trying to find her way through the maze of parenthood to be confronted with the inevitable onslaught of opinions from family, friends, and even strangers about how quickly a child should wean, where and how long a child should sleep, how often you should hold a baby, or how much separation parents should have from their newborn. I hope this book empowers you with the knowledge you need to not only trust yourself, but trust your baby as well.

THE BASICS OF BREASTFEEDING

From the outside looking in, the nuts and bolts of breastfeeding—latching and positioning—look as simple and instinctual as picking up your infant and placing him in front of your breast. However, those two small instinctive acts are where most breastfeeding problems begin. In this chapter, I will discuss how to achieve a perfect and pain-free latch, proper positioning of you and your baby, switching breasts, and the myriad breastfeeding accessories available to us now. Finally, I'll discuss the role of your support system in maintaining a healthy supply of milk.

LATCHING

A perfect latch is the jackpot of breastfeeding. Without one, breastfeeding can quickly lead to sore and painful nipples or even nipple cracks and bleeding. I'll talk extensively about infant anatomical abnormalities that can make latching difficult in Chapter 5 (see page 50), but for now let's examine what a great latch looks and feels like. In your quest for the perfect latch, you might feel a little tugging, a bit of pulling, and the faintest hint of soreness. Anything beyond these three feelings means that something might be wrong with your infant's latch. Ultimately, the perfect latch feels like nothing at all—a little bit of pressure, but mostly just you, your baby, and a rush of bonding hormones filling you with a sense of calm. If you feel anything beyond the mildest bit of soreness, you should have your baby's latch examined by a lactation consultant immediately. Above all else, nursing should not hurt.

Our anatomy is set up for infants to nurse without causing us pain. Your baby should not ever suck on your nipple; rather, suckling should take place on the areola—the dark region around your nipple. The nipple isn't designed to be sucked on with the power and force that it takes to effectively draw milk out of the breast. Even the smallest misstep in latching can cause pain and soreness for days. I understand these warnings can sound dire, but I assure you, the majority of infants come out of the womb ready to suckle properly and nurse immediately. If you're worried that you've never nursed a baby before, just remember that your little one has never nursed before either. So you two are in this thing together! You will figure it out in tandem, with the help of your support team.

The key to a perfect latch is for your baby to have a nice, big, open mouth that takes in a large portion of the areola. No two areolas are the same, and to make matters even more complicated, the darkened area of the areola typically grows quite large during pregnancy to help give infants a visual guide of where to go to eat. Essentially your areolas are like two big round signs that say "Eat Here!" in flashing neon lights. Depending on the size of your areola, your baby might get only a small portion of it in his mouth, and that's just fine. As long as he has a big, wide latch that isn't painful to you and transfers milk effectively, it is the perfect latch. As you can see, the perfect latch for one woman might not be the perfect latch for the next.

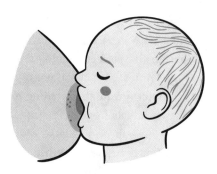

Good latch

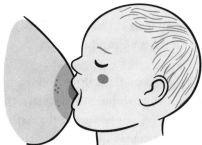

Bad latch

When your infant latches on properly and begins to suck, it triggers a hormonal reaction that allows your mammary glands to let milk flow freely and in large spurts. These are called "letdowns"; many women have described them as feeling like a great release or even sometimes a tingling sensation in their breast as they nurse. Some women will feel a letdown and some will not. But whether you feel it or not, it's happening. A series of letdowns is part of the natural cycle of a nursing session. You may notice that your infant begins to suck rapidly through these letdowns and then slows down when they're over or even appears to stop nursing altogether until another letdown happens. Letdowns tend to occur more frequently at the start of a nursing session and decrease as a nursing session continues, sometimes giving the appearance that your baby is asleep at the breast when he is, in fact, resting and waiting for the next letdown.

The perfect latch means there is optimal milk transfer. The amount your baby transfers in each nursing session will vary throughout the day, just like the amount of food you eat varies throughout the day. To learn how to evaluate your supply and find out if your baby is getting enough milk, see Chapter 4.

POSITIONING

Part of getting to the perfect latch is positioning the baby properly at the breast. Once again, *properly* and *perfect* are subjective terms, as it all depends on what feels good for you and your baby. There are many different nursing positions possible, and while it can be tempting in your quest to win the breastfeeding Olympics to try all of them, this isn't necessary. Once you find the position that works well for you and your baby, stick to it. It's important that this position promotes an effective latch for your baby and is one in which you're comfortable. Your body should be able to relax and withstand nights of cluster feedings or growth spurts that seem to never end (but always do). If any of the following happens while you are nursing, it's time to find a new position:

- You find that you're slumped forward or bent back
- You experience shoulder pain
- Your wrist starts to hurt
- Your arm "falls asleep"
- You experience back pain

These are all signs that, while nursing in this position might be working for your little one, it won't work for you in the long run. So what will? Six common and typically comfortable nursing positions are the cradle hold, cross-cradle hold, football hold, laid-back or biological nursing position, seated hold, and side-lying nursing.

Cradle and Cross-Cradle Positions

The cradle and cross-cradle positions are two of the most widely used positions. They are the natural ways in which we hold infants, cradled close to our bodies and held securely. In the cradle and cross-cradle position, you will want to sit up straight on a comfortable chair, couch, or bed—ideally, a seat without arms on it, so you can freely move your arms to position yourself and your baby better.

To nurse in the cross-cradle position, hold your baby with the opposite arm and hand from the breast you're feeding with by supporting the back of your baby's head with your open hand. If you need to support your breast, you can do so with your other hand. If you don't need to support your breast, then your other arm can either relax or go directly under the arm actively holding your little one.

The cradle position is very similar to the cross-cradle position, except the other arm is actively holding your baby. In the cradle position,

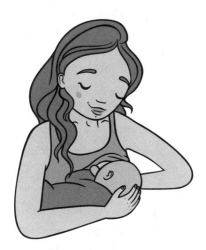

Cross-cradle position

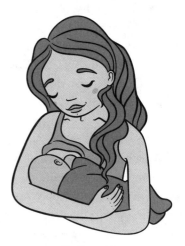

Cradle position

hold and support your baby with the arm on the same side of your body as the breast you're feeding with. So, if you're nursing on the left side, support your baby with your left arm, and if you are nursing on the right side, support your baby with your right arm. With the cradle position, instead of your baby's head resting on your open hand, it will now be resting in the crook of your arm. While this position can be a natural, easy way to nurse, one major pitfall can be your natural tendency to slouch forward to meet the baby to nurse. This can cause pain in your back, shoulders, arms, and wrists. Instead, in this position and all positions, you should bring your baby toward you to nurse, pulling him up and close to you rather than leaning toward him. Keep your baby in a neutral and comfortable position with your arms holding him securely, but stay relaxed. While it may be helpful for some mothers to hold their breast when nursing young infants who don't yet have the head, neck, and body control to stay at the breast effectively, it isn't necessary for all mothers to do this. If you and your infant can nurse comfortably without supporting your breast with your hands, then by all means do so.

Football Hold

The football hold is a favorite of hospital lactation consultants because it gives the breastfeeding mother a lot of control over her infant's position, especially if the baby is squirming or small and needs lots of support at the breast. It's also a great position for mothers who have had a cesarean section and mothers who have large or pendulous breasts. However, you should remember that just because it might be the favorite position of the lactation consultant who taught you to nurse at the hospital, this doesn't mean it has to be yours, or even that

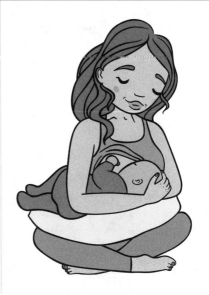

Football hold

you have to master this position. Remember, even when someone is showing you multiple nursing positions, you should always stick with the one that's the most comfortable for you and your baby. If the football hold isn't it, that's OK.

The name "football hold" comes from the position in which you're holding your baby—as if you were a quarterback running down the field with the ball tucked under your arm. Sit comfortably and position your baby on the side of your body that you'll be feeding from. Hold your little one close, with his abdomen touching the side of your rib cage. In the early stages, using a nursing pillow can be useful to help position your baby while you work on getting your arms and hands in the right place. With your open hand, support your baby's head and guide it toward your breast. If you need to support your breast, use the open hand from your inactive arm. This is also the most common position used to nurse two infants at once, although siblings can also comfortably be nursed while they're in a seated position or in two different positions at once, such as one infant in a cradle hold and the other in football hold.

Laid-Back Position

Much as the name "laid-back breastfeeding" implies, in this position all you have to do is lie back and your baby does the rest. Of course, you'll want to make sure that he's well supported by your hands, but in this position the baby calls the shots. Many now believe that the laid-back position is the most natural position for an infant to nurse in, which is why it also goes by the name "biological nurturing" or "biological nursing." In fact, immediately after birth, if allowed, an infant will slowly crawl on his own up his mother's stomach and to the breast of his choosing and latch on. Newborns are not known for their speed or accuracy, so this process can take anywhere from thirty

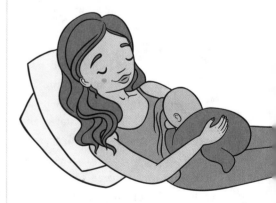

Laid-back position

minutes to an hour, which is why it's not often observed. However, seeing infants do this on their own is an awe-inspiring treat.

If you don't have the time to wait for your infant to crawl all the way up your belly to latch on his own, don't worry—there's a shortcut. In this position you'll need to position yourself comfortably in bed or on a sofa with an ottoman so that you're in a well-supported, reclined position. Position your little one on your stomach right in front of your breast so that you're stomach to stomach. He will do a lot of bobbing around at the breast, opening his mouth widely to take in the nipple and coming back up to correct his position and latch if he does not do it properly the first time. This position facilitates a wide latch that gives your baby complete control over the feeding process. If you have a strong or fast letdown reflex—the hormonal reaction that causes your milk to surge in a large stream—then this position allows your infant to let some milk fall out of his mouth rather than trying to suck it all down at a frantic pace. Laid-back nursing is a relaxing position in which you and your baby should be well supported and able to enjoy the experience of nursing together.

Seated Hold

The seated breastfeeding position is one that older babies who have good control over their heads and necks tend to naturally do on their own. Depending on the developmental stage, many infants will even go from sitting to standing at the breast in this position, straddling your legs. This position is also useful for mothers who have a strong or fast letdown or for infants with swallowing difficulties, physical anomalies (like a cleft palate), or problems with reflux. To breastfeed your baby in a seated position, sit him on one thigh, hugging him

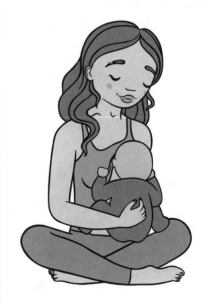

Seated hold

closely to your body. Support his back and head with your hand as needed according to his developmental stage.

Side-Lying Position

Side-lying is an ideal position for just about any time of day but is especially useful when your little one is going through a growth spurt and is nursing more often and longer than usual. Side-lying is a passive nursing position in which almost your entire body can relax, allowing you to nurse in comfort—making it an ideal nighttime nursing position as well. In fact, many mothers have told me that just the small act of lying down to nurse at night rather than sitting up in bed or in a chair makes a great deal of difference in how rested they feel the next day. To nurse in the side-lying position, lie on your side with your baby facing your breast. Support your little one with one hand and position your other arm above your head. This formation is a natural and instinctive position called the "Mother's C." You'll notice that with your little one lying next to you, your arm will automatically extend above your head and your knees will curl up to provide a cocoon for him to nurse in. This is a protective position that helps prevent rolling onto or away from your baby as well as prevents others nearby from doing the same.

SWITCHING BREASTS

Some women worry that they won't be able to adequately feed their baby due to the size of their breasts. However, you can't determine your breast milk storage capacity by looking at your breast. The size or shape does not determine how much milk each breast can hold at one time. A mother with a higher breast milk storage capacity has all the milk her infant needs for one nursing session in one breast, while a mother with a moderate breast milk storage capacity has all the milk her infant needs for one nursing session split between both breasts—neither is "right" or better. Sometimes your infant will nurse

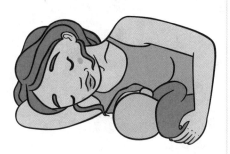

Side-lying position

at one breast, sometimes both. It all depends on your breasts' storage capacity, your infant's calorie needs at that time, or even your infant's mood at that nursing session.

How will you know when and if to switch breasts during a nursing session? Follow your infant's cues. If your infant nurses at one breast, then unlatches, content and no longer showing signs of hunger, then the nursing session is complete. If he nurses on one side but is still showing signs of hunger, then offer the other breast. Early signs of hunger in an infant include smacking lips, rooting, trying to get into a nursing position, suckling, or attempting to suck on his lips, fingers, or hands. However, not every infant will have these same hunger cues, and some of these are just normal baby behavior. For instance, in many babies, lip smacking isn't related to hunger, whereas in some infants it is. It's important to watch your baby's body language to learn what his needs are as best you can.

ENGORGEMENT

Engorgement of the breast occurs when colostrum is transitioning into mature milk and your milk volume dramatically increases, seemingly overnight (see Chapter 3 for more on the science behind making milk). This influx of mature milk pushes your breasts to their maximum capacity and causes pain, swelling, and a feeling of tightness in the breast. Engorgement can make the breast so hard and swollen that it can be difficult for your little one to latch. Many mothers find that using a warm compress (such as a warm, wet towel) applied before nursing along with a little hand expression can make nursing easier and help relieve some of the pain of engorgement.

While it can be tempting to pump when your breasts start to feel engorged, it is important that you resist that urge. During periods of engorgement your breasts are overreacting and making more milk than your infant needs. If you pump to relieve engorgement, you are signaling your body to not only continue to make milk but to make more milk, which will only make engorgement worse. The only way to tell your body to stop making so much milk is to allow your little one to nurse on demand. Your baby will tell your body exactly how much milk he needs. Within one to two days with a normal, on-demand nursing routine, engorgement subsides in most women.

If your engorgement symptoms last longer than two days, then it is time to reach out to an experienced health care practitioner to ensure that you are not suffering from symptoms of plugged ducts or mastitis and to an IBCLC to ensure that your infant's latch, positioning, and milk transfer are effective.

Even though breast engorgement is an inevitable part of the breastfeeding experience for most mothers within the first week postpartum, there are some things you can do to lessen the severity of your engorgement symptoms and help resolve them quickly:

- Nurse on demand (at least ten times a day in the early days of nursing).
- Watch your baby, not the clock. Allow your little one to nurse until he completely drains the breast.
- Have your little one's latch checked to ensure that he is transferring milk properly.
- Hand express while in the shower to help relieve tension and pain.

DO I NEED BREASTFEEDING ACCESSORIES?

At least 80 percent of my breastfeeding clients ask me if they should buy the new lactation cookie, tea, or supplement on the market. By and large, the answer is no. Unfortunately, all these products do is increase the myth of low milk supply (see Part II). Many mothers unnecessarily take fenugreek capsules, eat lactation cookies, and drink lactation teas before any supply issues even arise. One of the uniquely wonderful things about breastfeeding is that it doesn't require any gear, tests, or bells and whistles. Our modern world has brought us lots of fun helpers like breastfeeding pillows, nursing tank tops, and nursing pads. Ultimately, however, all the extra gear is just optional; women all around the world since the beginning of humanity have been able to effectively nurse their infants without the use of expensive tests and gear. Here's my take on how essential some common breastfeeding accessories are.

Breast Pump

Breast pumps have become a staple of the breastfeeding experience in the United States. Many hospitals will have a hospital-grade pump waiting for you in your hospital room shortly after birth. However, a breast pump is not a necessity for all mothers, and using a breast pump too soon can do more harm than good. Rest assured that until you are ready for your first separation from your little one, there is usually very little need to use a breast pump in the early weeks and months of nursing. In Chapter 6, I'll explore the ins and outs of using a breast pump, when to use one, and how to use one.

Nursing Pads

The key to getting motherhood right, if there is such a thing, is to not compare yourself to other mothers. Some mothers begin to leak colostrum weeks before their baby is born, while some never leak. Each woman in each scenario is normal. If you are a mother who is prone to leaking, it can be helpful to keep reusuable nursing pads on standby. Bamboo fiber or cotton pads tend to provide the best protection, while disposable pads can be handy while traveling. If you do find yourself needing a nursing pad, chances are you won't need one until your milk volume increases, which is not until three to seven days after the birth of your little one—so these aren't hospital-bag essentials but rather something nice to have around the house just in case.

At-Home Breast Milk Test

In addition to lactation supplements, smoothies, teas, and cookies, there's a growing market of tests and monitors designed specifically with the breastfeeding mother in mind. There are laboratory tests that analyze the nutritional content of your breast milk, at home tests that give an approximation of the amount of alcohol in your breast milk, and even shady tests that claim to be able to measure the exact volume of milk you have in each breast. While these tests are tempting to buy, they're unnecessary and can cause more anxiety than relief. Maternal alcohol intake being a threat to your baby is largely a myth, and even when the breastfeeding mother has a very nutrient-poor or low-caloric diet, the quality of nutrients in her breast milk typically remains high. Don't forget that breast milk is the only biological norm of nutrition for infants and that breast milk production is very forgiving!

The myths of having to "pump and dump" after consuming alcoholic beverages and of babies becoming "drunk" after mom has a glass or two of wine are still pervasive. But I assure you, they are just myths. Very little alcohol passes directly into the breast milk, and when it does it's usually cycled out of the milk within two hours. If you have a glass of wine or a cocktail right after nursing your little one, by the time he is ready to nurse again, it's likely that your breast milk is clear of alcohol. The general rule of alcohol consumption and breastfeeding is that if you feel good enough to parent, then you're probably in good shape to breastfeed. If you're feeling lethargic or dizzy or are unable to hold your baby, then it's wise to wait until you have sobered up a bit before nursing. Offer your little one a bottle of previously expressed breast milk, then pump and dump to maintain supply until you're feeling up to par again.

Nursing Pillow

Nursing pillows have become the must-have gift at baby showers and a ubiquitous part of the Western nursing experience. While nursing pillows are a lovely creature comfort and can make nursing in the first few weeks more comfortable, they aren't a necessary part of the nursing experience and certainly have their own set of downsides. Nursing pillows are, by design, typically not deep enough for most mothers to nurse effectively with just one pillow. Many mothers find themselves slouched over in the cradle, cross-cradle, or football-hold position, attempting to bring their breast down to the level of the pillow. This, inevitably, causes back and shoulder pain. So, if you're using a nursing pillow, always support it with another pillow or a rolled-up/folded blanket to prevent slouching. You can also ditch the nursing pillow altogether and just use a couple of regular bed pillows as support. Infants grow quickly and therefore outgrow nursing pillows fast. Typically, by eight to twelve weeks of age, most infants have grown too big for their nursing pillows.

Nursing Bra/Tank/Gown

Nursing bras can be handy for nursing mothers since they have snaps on the top of each cup that fold down to allow easy access to the breast for nursing. While nursing bras are nice to have, they aren't a necessity. Any well-fitting bra can work for breastfeeding as long as it doesn't constrict your breasts. Choose a front-closure bra if you want to be able to just unsnap it open for your little one to nurse. Otherwise, simply lift up your bra to allow him access.

Although also not 100 percent necessary, nursing tank tops and gowns can be nice to have. Many women find that using a nursing tank instead of a nursing bra is helpful, especially when nursing in public. Depending on the type of shirt you're wearing, when nursing in public your abdomen may be exposed for a short period of time while adjusting your baby. If this makes you feel uncomfortable, use a nursing tank under your shirt, so that your abdomen is never exposed while nursing in public. Nursing gowns, meanwhile, are a good nighttime option if you already sleep in a nightgown. Though these acessories can be nice, when it comes to nursing at home, there are no rules: Go braless, wear a sleeping bra, wear a comfortable bra of your choosing—it is completely up to you.

A properly fitting bra is incredibly important to a positive breastfeeding experience. Although you don't necessarily need a nursing bra or tank, you do need a bra that fits your cup size to ensure that your breasts aren't being constricted and that your milk ducts don't become blocked due to pinching from your bra. Especially because cup sizes will change during pregnancy and after childbirth, consider getting fitted for a bra at the lingerie store or department to be sure you're wearing the right size.

You also want a bra that doesn't compress your breasts—sports bras are an excellent example of bras that constrict your breasts and can lead to a decrease in milk supply. As long as your bra fits properly, it can have underwire, although many women choose to not use bras with underwire, as the risk for breast compression or pinching of milk ducts is higher.

Nipple Cream

Before my daughter was born, many of my friends told me to buy cases of lanolin-based nipple cream to help with the first few weeks of nursing. This kind of advice is par for the course for new mothers when it comes to nursing. The expectation is that nursing is going to hurt, so do all you can to be prepared for the pain, including buying various types of nipple creams and butters. However, this is simply untrue. If nursing hurts in any way, then it's time to have your little one's latch and positioning looked at immediately, so you can adjust it to make nursing more comfortable. While lanolin-based products can be a big help for mothers who have nipple soreness, you don't necessarily have to go out and purchase a cream or butter made specifically for nursing mothers. I've seen half-ounce jars of nipple butter for over twenty dollars! Frankly, this is just a waste of money. A little coconut oil or even olive oil can do the same job as store-bought nipple creams and often for a fraction of the price.

Formula

When you get those little samples of formula that nearly every mother receives in the mail or at the doctor's office, well-meaning friends, family members, and even health care professionals will tell you to keep them "just in case." While this may seem like sound advice, especially in light of all the tough times and horror stories you've heard about breastfeeding, it's actually one of the first of many subtle ways in which a mother's confidence in her ability to nurse is undermined. Dozens of studies from around the world examining mothers of all ethnicities, age groups, and education levels have all shown that a mother's confidence in her ability to breastfeed is one of the greatest predictors of successful breastfeeding.[1] And in my own private practice, I've found that if a mother keeps formula in the home, she will end up using it eventually—especially in the absence of good breastfeeding support and education. For this reason, I recommend that you keep formula out of your home—even the free samples! There are evidenced-based protocols and guidelines in place for the appropriate use of formula as a supplement both inside and outside of a hospital setting (which I will discuss more in depth on page 63).

SUPPORT

Sometimes as a parent you're a rock star. You're the mom at the grocery store or mall making parenthood look easy. Saying and doing all the right things, soothing your baby in just the way he needs—you have it all under control. But sometimes everything that can go wrong does so simultaneously. You're exhausted beyond words, you can't put two sentences together, and if anyone so much as looks at you sympathetically, you might burst into tears. You don't want to be touched anymore, and you can't stand the feeling of those little hands exploring your body as your little one nurses. You just need a break! You need some help, and you need it right now. In those moments, if someone tells you "They're only a baby once!" or "It goes by so fast!" your first instinct is likely to punch them in the nose and scream. In those moments, you need your mommy tribe, you need support, and you need someone to vent to who will just let you get it all out.

Having supportive family, friends, and community is as essential to successfully nursing your infant as building and maintaining a healthy milk supply. Parenthood is a journey that no one makes on their own, and breastfeeding is an important part of that journey for the entire family— not just mother and baby. Having a solid support team around you is just as important as (if not more important than) anything else you could learn in this book.

One of my mentors would always tell new mothers in her La Leche League support group that a mother should be in bed for the first six weeks after giving birth, on the couch for the next six weeks, and then up and about for the following six weeks. While this advice might not work for mothers who have a limited amount of time away from work, it does start a great conversation about how a mother should spend the precious time she does have with her little one at home.

One of the principal jobs of your support team should be to help you manage stress. Stress plays a major role in a mother's ability to make and transfer milk to her infant (see more about this on page 85), and one of the greatest challenges for a new mother is balancing motherhood with an endless sea of family and friends excited to meet the new addition to the family. It's hard enough to acclimate to all the new demands of parenthood without everyone you love and respect watching your every move! So as friends and family sojourn to your house to meet your new baby, don't be afraid to put them to good use. So many people will ask you what they can do for you or if you need anything. This is the time to speak up and say yes. Don't be afraid to ask your guests if they can grab some take-out for you on the way to your house, or throw a load of laundry into the dryer for you. If it's been a while since you've had a decent shower, or a shower at all, nurse your little one and then use the time with another adult in the house to grab a few moments for yourself. Take care of yourself and allow others to take care of you, too.

THE SCIENCE BEHIND MAKING MILK

Now that you know what you need to know to properly breastfeed, you might be wondering . . . how is all of this happening? After all, for many women, days before the double pink lines on a pregnancy test tell them they are pregnant, their breasts have already begun to give them clues that something in their body is changing. For some it's a little tenderness, for others a slight tingling sensation. But for nearly all mothers-to-be, from the moment of conception, the body is already setting out on the task of making milk for the baby. At just twelve weeks of pregnancy, your body has begun to more fully develop the ducts and glands that will form the building blocks of milk production. The first stage of milk production starts a little before the midpoint of your pregnancy,[1] which means that for the majority of your pregnancy there's already enough milk in your breasts to feed your infant at birth.

Before I go on to discuss some of the reasons why a woman might experience low milk supply, let me first give you an overview of the various stages of milk production and the hormones that control them. These hormones aren't dependent on your age or biological connection to your infant. Whether you're twenty-five or forty-five, conceived naturally, used an egg donor, or are a surrogate, your body will begin to make these hormonal shifts and changes as soon as the baby is born and the placenta is delivered.

THE STAGES OF MILK PRODUCTION

The multifaceted process by which the body creates milk is called "lactogenesis." It's a sensitive process dependent on pharmacological, physical, and psychological influences that affect each step in the process. Lactogenesis consists of three steps, lactogenesis I through III.

Lactogenesis I, the first step, begins in pregnancy and is partially brought about by a sharp increase in your body's serum prolactin levels—up to twenty times higher than their prepregnancy levels (more about prolactin in a minute). In the second trimester of pregnancy, your body begins to make a type of milk called colostrum. Colostrum is a powerhouse of nutrition and immunity for your newborn. It's a complete food providing all the protein, fat, carbohydrates, vitamins, and minerals your infant needs in a compact serving size of half to two teaspoons per feeding.

There are thousands of components that make up colostrum. On the next page is a sampling of the nutrient and immune compounds found in colostrum and their functions.

The hormonal changes of birth cause colostrum to rapidly change into mature milk, and lactogenesis II begins approximately one to three days postpartum, with most mothers noting a sharp increase in milk volume between days four to seven postpartum.[2] Lactogenesis II is what is commonly referred to as a mother's milk "coming in." However, prior to lactogenesis II, you are making milk (colostrum) that's appropriate in volume and nutrient composition for your baby.

During lactogenesis I and II, your milk supply is completely regulated by hormones. However, once lactogenesis III begins around twelve weeks postpartum, it's now your baby's job to ensure that your milk supply stays steady and meets her demands. This means that if your baby doesn't nurse, your body won't make milk; the more your little one nurses, the more milk you will make. For mothers whose milk supply begins to decrease seemingly overnight, this is often the culprit. If you're one of these mothers, you may have initially had a very high milk supply and an infant who had a poor ability to suck and transfer milk at the breast. The infant's suck was never a productive one—the latch and suction at the breast were

COLOSTRUM COMPONENT[3]	FUNCTION
Lactoferrin	An antimicrobial component of breast milk and colostrum that actively attacks harmful bacteria and fungi (including *E. coli* and salmonella); also has anti-inflammatory properties and helps transfer iron to the blood cells; some studies have also shown it has antiviral properties.
Lactoperoxidase	An antibacterial enzyme that protects against infection; has also shown antiviral activity toward some viruses, in particular the polioviruses.
Immunoglobulin A (IgA)	Primarily resides in the gastrointestinal tract, respiratory tract, and urogenital tract and prevents negative pathogens from colonizing (growing).
Immunoglobulin G (IgG)	Provides immune defense from harmful pathogens and plays an integral role in overall immunity.
Immunoglobulin M (IgM)	Antibodies that are the body's first responders to harmful pathogens.
Immunoglobulin D (IgD)	Helps the body create specific antibodies for invading pathogens.
Epidermal growth factor (EGF)	Regulates cell growth in the skin, gut, and mammary glands.
Transforming growth factor alpha (TGF-α)	Encourages epithelial tissue growth.
Transforming growth factor beta (TGF-β)	Crucial to tissue regeneration, regulation of the immune system, and formation of cartilage.
Insulin-like growth factor 1 (IGF-1)	Plays an integral role in infant and childhood growth and development.
Growth hormone (GH)	Regulates a variety of cellular functions including cell growth and development.
Cytokines	An important part of cellular communication; help regulate growth and development and contribute to controlling the body's inflammatory response.

not correct—but because you had a larger-than-typical milk volume, the baby was able to transfer milk without working to do so. So while the baby appeared to be nursing, she was simply drinking and not actively stimulating your breast to continue to make milk.

MILK-MAKING HORMONES

The majority of hormones involved in breast milk production are housed in the pituitary gland, a pea-sized gland in your brain tucked away neatly behind the bridge of your nose. Your hormones work hard all day carrying messages around your body telling each system how to function and cooperate, and this tiny little gland is home base for most of them. It's divided into two parts—the anterior pituitary and the posterior pituitary. The anterior pituitary produces adrenocorticotrophic hormones (ACTH), thyroid-stimulating hormones (TSH), luteinizing hormones (LH), follicle-stimulating homones (FSH), prolactin, growth hormones, and melanocyte-stimulating hormones (MSH). Your posterior pituitary gland produces antidiuretic hormones (ADH) and oxytocin. In understanding the reasons for low milk supply, it's important to understand how these hormones affect breast milk production.

Prolactin

The primary function of prolactin is to stimulate the breast to make milk. Prolactin levels in the body are at their highest during pregnancy and the first months of breastfeeding. The majority of lactogenic foods, herbs, and medications used today and for thousands of years work by increasing the amount of prolactin synthesized, stored, and released by the body. The anterior pituitary houses prolactin, and therefore any disruption or disease that affects the anterior pituitary will likely have a negative impact on lactation. Prolactin does not function alone in the body. Instead, it's part of a complex system of nursing hormones including oxytocin, serotonin, and dopamine.[4]

Upon the onset of lactogenesis II, prolactin is released in response to suckling or the simulated sucking of a breast pump or hand expression. A series of nerves and receptors carries this suckling response to the brain through the spinal nerves of the C8 to T2 vertebrae, in the upper back—oxytocin also travels this same route.[5] Interestingly, several case studies have demonstrated that adjustments of the spinal column by a chiropractor can help prolactin travel unobstructed from its stimulus point in the areola to the brain,[6] enabling milk production.

Oxytocin

Oxytocin is affectionately referred to as the love hormone. A rush of oxytocin will not only make two people adore each another, it can make them more trusting, lessen fears, and reduce anxiety.[7] Overall, it's the hormone that keeps you happy, calm, and in love. With this in mind, it should come as no surprise that your body releases massive quantities of oxytocin the moment your child is born, as well as every single time she nurses.[8] The bonding experience that mothers report having with their infants while nursing is, predominantly, a hormonally mediated one. Many mothers report feeling sleepy when they breastfeed; this sensation of calm and sleepiness is directly related to oxytocin. By releasing this powerful hormone, your body is doing all it can to reduce your anxiety and stress so you can focus simply on loving and caring for your precious little one every time you nurse.

Cortisol

The adrenal glands produce a variety of hormones related to our "fight or flight" reflexes and how our bodies respond to stressors, and cortisol is one of them.

ACTH, which is produced in the pituitary gland, stimulates the adrenal gland to make cortisol. Medical conditions that affect the anterior pituitary gland (such as Cushing's disease) can also influence the way our body synthesizes cortisol.

Cortisol helps control some of the body's most important functions, including blood pressure, blood sugar levels, and metabolism. It also has anti-inflammatory properties and provides resistance to stress in the body. In terms of lactation, cortisol facilitates the binding of prolactin to mammary receptors.[9] Pregnancy, childbirth, and parenthood are full of natural stressors, and cortisol works to help your body cope with them and allows prolactin to easily do its job of making milk without interruption. In animal studies in which both cortisol and prolactin were given to animals, milk supply increased dramatically.[10] However, this does not mean that cortisol supplements should be used to increase milk production. While cortisol plays an important role in breast milk production and stress reduction, there are currently no human studies that have shown a benefit to using cortisol supplements or cortisol stimulating medications to increase milk production.

PART TWO

The Myth of Low Milk Supply:

SEPARATING FACT FROM FICTION

AM I EXPERIENCING LOW MILK SUPPLY OR TRANSFER?

The first moment that a mother puts her baby to her breast is often filled with an undercurrent of anxiety. Will breastfeeding hurt? Will I have enough milk? This is an anxiety whose seeds were likely planted decades earlier, before she even thought about having a child or breastfeeding. If you feel any pain when you're nursing, I urge you to find an International Board Certified Lactation Consultant in your area to have you and your baby evaluated. Above all else, nursing should not hurt. You shouldn't wince in pain every time your infant latches or hesitate before putting him to your breast because you know that toe-curling pain is around the corner. Ultimately, nursing should feel like nothing more than a small tug with the occasional rush of oxytocin giving you a calm, happy feeling while nursing your baby.

Aside from pain, typically, a mother's next concern is her milk supply. Agalactorrhea, the medical term for having a low milk supply, is a rare condition only seen in approximately 1 percent of the world's population. I'll go into some of the reasons behind this condition in Chapter 5, and some of the nonmedical reasons you might be experiencing a low milk supply in Chapter 6, but first, let's start with the basics: evaluating your supply, making sure your infant is getting enough nutrients, and deciding what to do next.

Milk supply and milk transfer are two interlinked but different concepts. A mother's milk supply is the amount of milk she's presently making for her infant, while milk transfer is the amount of milk an infant consumes during each nursing session. Figuring out if you're making enough milk and if your baby is transferring enough milk is relatively straightforward, but there are a lot of old wives' tales and misinformation about signs of low milk supply and improper milk transfer.

EVALUATING YOUR MILK SUPPLY

Throughout your breastfeeding journey, your body will make milk based on the needs of your child. The cycle of making milk is based on demand and supply. Essentially, as your child begins to nurse more and "demand" more milk from you, your body will rise to the task and make not only enough milk for your little one, but also an extra ounce or so as a "just in case" reserve.

In the era of social media, we're in the unique position of easily being able to lean on our village of parents to help get us through the hardest moments of parenthood as well as to share our triumphs. But while having the support of other parents is invaluable when taking on the task of raising tiny humans, it's important that in doing so, you don't begin to compare yourself with other parents, especially when it comes to your milk supply. One mother might post her "stash" of five hundred ounces tucked away in her freezer, while another may share her struggle of only being able to pump two to four ounces total in a single pumping session. Before you get caught up in it all, remember: Often, mothers who have a large stash of breast milk in the freezer either have oversupply, which carries with it its own risk and challenges, or they're exclusively pumping around the clock for an infant who can't yet feed at the breast for a variety of reasons. Additionally, some mothers simply respond to the pump better than others. A breast pump removes milk from the breast by pulling directly on the nipple using vacuum suction, whereas a baby massages the areola gently to remove milk. For most mothers, a massage is a much more pleasant method of milk removal than a mechanical vacuum pull.

Breast pumps are a relatively new phenomenon in breastfeeding history. The first breast pump was patented in the mid-nineteenth century. Back then, the purpose of the pump wasn't to express milk but to help pull out inverted nipples to make breastfeeding easier for affected women.[1] It wasn't until 1991 that the first electric breast pump was sold commercially. When the first commercial-grade electric breast pumps became available, the widely held belief was that mothers should use breast pumps to measure and assess the volume of breast milk they were making and providing for their infants. To this day, many practitioners still urge mothers to use a breast pump to evaluate their milk supply. However, breast pumps don't remove milk from the breast as effectively as an infant does, which means that, in general, a mother will pump less milk than her body is actually producing. (See page 75 about getting more milk out of pumping).

Normal output from expressing milk via an electric breast pump is typically a half ounce to two ounces total. If you're currently pumping and getting anything in this range, rest assured that you're normal and this output is normal. For mothers who are exclusively pumping, pumping two to four ounces total in a pumping session is normal.

Because mothers who are exclusively breastfeeding might have an output of a half ounce to two ounces, it's also normal for it to take multiple pumping sessions to fill one three-ounce bottle for an infant.

So, when is the right time to start pumping? I suggest beginning about two weeks before you return to work or school, have your first girls' night out since your baby was born, or go on a a baby-free date night. Milk volume is typically the highest in the morning, which makes it a good time to experiment with pumping for the first time. After your first two morning nursing sessions, you can try pumping for ten to fifteen minutes to see how your body responds to the pump. Remember, this won't give you an accurate picture of how much milk you're making, especially if pumping after a nursing session. This is just an opportunity to get used to the mechanics of pumping and to start putting a little milk away in the refrigerator or freezer in preparation for your infant's first bottle. While having a large stash of breast milk in the freezer might feel good, it isn't a necessary part of the breastfeeding experience.

If you can manage to do so, it's good to pump enough extra milk for twenty-four hours of feeding and keep it on hand in the freezer in case there's an emergency and you and your infant are separated. While this is *nice* to have, it's not necessary, so don't let this be a point of parenting stress for you on your breastfeeding journey. Rest assured, if your baby is growing and developing normally and has an appropriate number of wet and soiled diapers (more on that in a minute), you're making enough milk.

IS MY BABY GETTING ENOUGH MILK?

A mother can have an excellent milk supply, even an oversupply, but if her infant doesn't have the ability to properly transfer that milk from the breast by suckling, then he'll become malnourished, and her milk supply will begin to decrease. An infant can have an ineffective suck for a variety reasons, from a tongue-tie to a lack of muscle tone due to premature birth, all of which I'll discuss later in Part II. But for now, let's look more closely at how to tell if your baby is getting enough milk.

Many mothers worry that if their infants are only nursing from one breast each session or don't nurse for long enough, they aren't getting enough milk. However, infant nursing patterns are highly variable and dependent on a number of factors. While you can find general guidelines for infant nursing behavior easily online, they are just that: general. Every infant is different, every mother is different, and every nursing session is different. Your milk changes from morning to night, from Friday to Monday. You and your baby are in a constant dance with his needs constantly evolving as he grows and your body rising to meet these changes and needs. On the next page is a table with the average reported intake of breast milk in infants. You will notice that the range of normal is very wide. After milk volume increases, somewhere between day four to seven postpartum, infants typically experience a small growth spurt. Your baby's milk intake can vary depending on when your milk volume increases and your baby's birth weight. Additionally, another growth spurt occurs around three weeks, which leads to wide variations in milk intake.

In general, a "normal" nursing session lasts anywhere from fifteen to sixty minutes and an infant will nurse every one to three hours.

INFANT AGE	INTAKE (ML/FEEDING, WITH 8 TO 12 FEEDINGS A DAY)[2]
24 hours or fewer	2–10
24–48 hours	5–15
48–72 hours	15–30
72–96 hours	30–60
1 week	45–60
1–6 months	70–112
7 months+	80–120

In cases where a mother has an oversupply and the infant has a very effective suck, the infant might transfer all he needs in a five-minute nursing session. At night when a mother's letdown isn't as fast and her milk volume has slightly decreased, the same infant might nurse for forty-five minutes. During a growth spurt, an infant who once nursed every two to three hours like clockwork might begin to nurse every hour! There's a wide variation of "normal" in your infant's world. If you're concerned about your infant's nursing patterns, then please reach

out to an International Board Certified Lactation Consultant for guidance. An IBCLC can help determine if your infant is transferring effectively and help you assess your infant's feeding cues between feedings and during a nursing session.

You may notice that health care practitioners seem to constantly ask how often your infant is urinating or passing bowel movements. Upon leaving the hospital, new parents are often given handouts with a guide to how many wet and poopy diapers they should see in a twenty-four-hour period and are encouraged to keep track of them. These numbers are important because they give you and your health care practitioner a good idea of how well nourished your infant is. The number of wet diapers he has in a day lets you know how hydrated your baby is, and the number of bowel movements lets you know how well nourished he is. The first sign that your infant is getting enough milk is that his diaper counts are on track. On the next page is a guide to how many wet and poopy diapers your infant should have in a twenty-four-hour period. If you're using disposable diapers, keep in mind that they are very absorbent, and many times an infant can urinate two to three times before you

INFANT AGE	IDEAL NUMBER OF WET DIAPERS	IDEAL NUMBER OF SOILED DIAPERS
1 day	1	1–2
2 days	2	1–2
3 days	3	3
4 days	4	3
5 days	5	3
6 days	6	3
7 or more days	6	3

notice it's wet. This chart counts one urination as one wet diaper.

If your little one is not presently meeting his diaper count goals—don't panic. Remember that diaper counts are just one measurement tool used to evaluate milk supply. Instead, reach out to your health care practitioner to help you evaluate your infant's overall health and growth and build a plan from there. While diaper counts are the best way for parents to tell if their child is getting enough milk, the most reliable way for a health practitioner to tell is by weight gain. If your health care provider has concerns about your infant's weight, she will typically have you come in for periodic weight checks. Immediately after birth, it's normal for infants to lose up to 10 percent of their initial body weight,[3] or even more for babies whose mothers were on an IV for any amount of time during their labor.[4] Many guidelines currently state that weight loss over 7 percent is undesirable; however, this percentage is based on babies who were fed formula only and doesn't take into account the well-documented variations in growth between breast-fed and formula-fed babies.[5] Most infants will regain their birth weight by two weeks of age, although some will take a little longer and some will gain weight more quickly. Unless you're directed to do so by your child's health care provider, I strongly advise against weighing your infant at home unless you're using a high-quality rented hospital scale, and the same scale each time, as there's a small yet incredibly important variation of approximately one to two ounces from scale to scale. Normal infant growth is a half ounce to one ounce a day. Sometimes an infant will go two to three days without growth and then grow three ounces in a day. This is why daily weigh-ins will not provide the most accurate assessment of milk transfer. Additionally, weighing an infant daily or multiple times a day can oftentimes create a high-stress situation for parents in which they are constantly watching the scale and not their infant. That's why, instead of weighing your infant at home, I recommend visiting a physician and looking at weight-gain trends such as the growth curve charts provided by the World Health Organization (WHO), which is one of the best ways to assess infant growth over the short and long term (you can find the WHO growth charts at cdc.gov/growthcharts/who_charts .htm).

MEDICAL REASONS FOR LOW MILK SUPPLY

Most mothers who believe they are struggling with a low milk supply due to medical or biological reasons are actually just experiencing a natural milk slump or other (nonmedical) breastfeeding issues. Only around 1 percent of women worldwide have true low-milk supply, which is typically caused by an underlying medical condition. Following are the predominant medical conditions affecting both mothers and babies that lead to true low milk supply. It's important to remember, however, that in most cases, even a mother who has medical reasons for low milk supply can provide some breast milk to her baby, just not enough to completely sustain her at the breast alone. Traditionally, other mothers from the community would come to the aid of a mother struggling with low milk supply and help take on the duties of feeding the infant by wet-nursing. While this practice isn't as popular in Western countries as in the rest of the world, there's a growing acceptance of using donor breast milk in its safest form, collected by local milk banks and laboratory tested and pasteurized to ensure safety.

BREAST REDUCTION SURGERY

Nearly all breast reduction surgeries (mammaplasties) are likely to decrease a woman's ability to breastfeed. Unfortunately, during breast reduction surgery, damage to the nerves, milk ducts, and alveoli (sacs of the mammary glands) is common. Depending on the way the surgery was done, some women might not be able to make enough milk, while others, because of the placement of the nipple after surgery, might not be able to get the milk from the milk ducts to the nipple. Many women are able to successfully breastfeed after mammaplasty, although supplementation is often necessary at some point.[1] It's important to note that although mammaplasty does have a potentially negative affect on breastfeeding, breast augmentation surgery (getting breast implants) does not typically have a negative effect on breastfeeding. The majority of women with a history of breast augmentation surgery are able to breastfeed exclusively.

If you have had breast reduction surgery in the past, contact an International Board Certified Lactation Consultant, preferably while you're pregnant, to go over your options and have a feeding plan in place to optimize the amount of milk you can produce. While breast reduction surgery does raise the risk that you will not be able to exclusively breastfeed your little one, it does not guarantee it. I have worked with many women in my clinical practice who were able to exclusively breastfeed after breast reduction surgery.

MASTITIS AND PLUGGED DUCTS

Breastfeeding brings about a series of expected and unexpected changes in the breast. Many times, it can be hard to discern the difference between the normal changes that occur during pregnancy and breastfeeding versus a sign that a serious problem is brewing. Plugged ducts often present as hard lumps in the breast, often at the base of the breast near the ribs, unlike engorgement, which causes the entire breast to swell and become hard to the touch. Plugged ducts are localized to one or more regions of the breast but typically do not affect the entire breast.

Plugged ducts can cause a temporary dip in your milk supply as the milk duct is physically blocked from allowing milk to flow freely from your breast to your baby. The best way to unclog a plugged duct is to nurse your baby frequently on the affected breast, massaging the breast as you nurse in the affected area to encourage milk flow. If your infant has an ineffective suck, then utilizing a breast pump can be helpful in clearing the plugged duct. Many mothers also find that taking an emulsifier like soy or sunflower helps to clear plugged ducts when used in combination with effective milk expression or nursing. A daily dose of 1,200 mg three or four times a day has been shown to help prevent and treat plugged ducts.[2]

Mastitis is the inflammation or infection of breast tissue, usually near a plugged duct. Most cases of mastitis occur within the first twelve weeks of breastfeeding when fluctuations in milk supply are the greatest. About 10 percent of breastfeeding women will develop mastitis sometime during their breastfeeding journey.[3] The most common cause of mastitis is inflammation or infection of a plugged duct due to inefficient milk removal. Mothers who have an infant with an ineffective suck or who are restricting the duration or frequency of feedings are at the highest risk for developing mastitis; additionally, mothers who have an oversupply of breastmilk are at a higher risk.[4]

Symptoms of mastitis include all the symptoms associated with plugged ducts, but with the addition of feelings of tenderness and heat at the site of the plugged duct,

redness, swelling, and a low-grade fever (101.3°F/38.5°C). Many mothers report feeling as if they have the flu with symptoms including aches, pain, and chills.

Women who consume a high-salt or high-fat diet may have a greater risk of developing mastitis. In animal studies, the risk of mastitis was higher in cows who had diets low in antioxidants, vitamin E, vitamin A, and selenium. However, human studies are inconclusive at this time and don't yet give us a clear picture of the nutritional causes, if any, behind mastitis.

One complication of mastitis is the development of breast abscesses. However, some abscesses are spontaneous and happen with or without the presence of mastitis. Abscesses are rare, only occurring in about 3 percent of women who develop mastitis; however, they mimic the symptoms of mastitis, including redness, swelling, and the area feeling warm to the touch.[5]

While you can, and in most cases should, still nurse through a plugged duct, mastitis, and even a breast abscess, your milk supply might take a hit while you are recovering from any of these conditions. Plugged ducts, mastitis, and breast abscesses, for the most part, are preventable. Frequent removal of milk from the breast by your baby is the number one way to reduce your risk of developing plugged ducts and mastitis. Additional factors that have been linked to plugged ducts and mastitis are stress, tight-fitting bras, using a manual breast pump, and nipple pain.[6]

Treatment of mastitis varies based on your symptoms; therefore it is paramount if you are experiencing any symptoms of mastitis or plugged ducts that you reach out to your health care provider for assistance, proper diagnosis, and treatment. Making sure you get enough rest (as much rest as one can with a newborn baby), drinking plenty of fluids, and eating a balanced diet are important to the healing process. Just as with plugged ducts, applying a warm compress or heat pack to the infected area prior to a feeding can facilitate a more productive milk flow, as well as compressing the breast throughout a nursing session to encourage milk flow. Some women will require antibiotics to treat mastitis. Treatment with antibiotics does increase your risk of thrush (a yeast infection of the skin). Symptoms of thrush are a constant burning pain in the breast and/or nipple and radiating pain throughout the breast that is also nearly constant. If you are experiencing these symptoms, it is imperative you and your infant see a health care provider immediately for proper treatment.

INSUFFICIENT GLANDULAR TISSUE

The causes of insufficient glandular tissue of the breast are varied. Congenital malformation is the leading known cause, with mothers who were born prematurely themselves being at the highest risk. However, disruption of growth and sex hormones during puberty (which can happen if you received hormonal treatment or had an eating disorder during your teen years, for example) can also cause insufficient glandular tissue development.

While your first instinct might be to wonder if small breasts are more likely to have insufficient glandular tissue development, this isn't the case. Insufficient tissue development can happen regardless of breast size. Although the primary function of our breasts is to make milk for our young, breast size is more complex than simply our milk-making capacity. Additionally, it's important to note that it's normal for one breast to be larger than the other, and/or for one breast to produce more milk than the other (irrespective of size). These aren't signs of insufficient glandular tissue development of the breast.

Insufficient glandular tissue development of the breast is rare. The initial sign is a lack of breast changes or growth throughout pregnancy. Lack of postpartum breast engorgement can also be a sign of insufficient glandular tissue development for some. However, breast engorgement is dependent on several factors, including the use of IV fluids during labor; therefore, it shouldn't be used as the only marker of insufficient glandular tissue. If you suspect that insufficient glandular tissue is the cause for your struggles with breastfeeding, seek out a definitive answer via a trained breast specialist or breast surgeon.

Even with underdeveloped breast tissue, most women can still breastfeed. In case reports on breastfeeding mothers with insufficient glandular tissue development of the breast, supplementation with formula or donor milk was necessary, but most women continued to nurse with the help of a supplemental nursing system or complementary breast- and bottle-feeding.[7]

POLYCYSTIC OVARY SYNDROME (PCOS)

Polycystic ovary syndrome (PCOS) is the most common reproductive disorder in women. It's estimated that anywhere from 3 to 15 percent of all women are affected by PCOS.[8] PCOS typically develops during puberty; however, there's new evidence that shows that substantial weight gain during your peak reproductive years can also lead to the development of PCOS.[9]

Symptoms of PCOS include irregular periods, cysts on the ovaries, and elevated androgen levels. There is an increased risk of infertility, development of type 2 diabetes, high cholesterol, metabolic syndrome, sleep apnea, and depression or anxiety in women with PCOS.

PCOS's effects on breastfeeding begin in the teen years as breasts are developing, likely far before a woman has even thought about becoming a mother. Elevated levels of androgens (male sex hormones like testosterone) in the body due to PCOS tend to decrease the amount of circulating estrogen and progesterone and can lead to insufficient glandular breast tissue development during puberty. Studies have even found that high levels of androgens appear to cause the breast to atrophy.[10] Women with high levels of androgens throughout pregnancy and immediately postpartum also tend to have problems with low milk supply. In fact, androgens have been traditionally used to rapidly inhibit lactation in mothers who didn't wish to continue breastfeeding.

If you have PCOS, you should have your androgen levels tested throughout pregnancy and the immediate postpartum period, as well as note any breast changes that occur during pregnancy—if you don't experience any changes at all, this could be a sign that your breast tissue didn't properly develop earlier in life. It's important to seek help from a lactation consultant prior to giving birth to create a postpartum feeding plan that takes into account your health history and current lab results. While androgens do have a negative effect on breastfeeding, not all women with PCOS will have high levels of androgens during pregnancy and the immediate postpartum period, and not all women with PCOS will have trouble breastfeeding due to low milk supply or delayed lactogenesis I or II. For those who do, eating galactagogues (foods that increase milk production; see page 104) and taking certain medications commonly used

to treat PCOS, such as metformin, can be helpful tools to increase the likelihood that breastfeeding will be successful.

THYROID ISSUES

Thyroid hormones are important for the expression of prolactin in lactating women. The thyroid hormone T4 (thyroxine) helps prolactin exert its milk-making powers, and during the prenatal period the number of thyroid hormone receptors in the mammary glands increases.[11] The issues of an underactive thyroid (hypothyroidism) and overactive thyroid (hyperthyroidism) can have a wide range of causes, some of which are directly related to pregnancy. The symptoms of both hypo- and hyperthyroidism can be tough to spot, since many of them are nearly indistinguishable from the symptoms of early motherhood!

Postpartum Hypothyroidism

Hypothyroidism occurs when your thyroid is making low levels of the hormone thyroxine. Symptoms include fatigue, weight gain, joint and muscle aches, thinning hair, decreased heart rate, depression, and impaired memory. Hypothyroidism can be caused by a variety of issues, including iodine deficiency, medications, pituitary disorders, and radiation therapy. Postpartum hypothyroidism most often occurs when your body produces antibodies against your own thyroid, causing your body to attack the thyroid and decrease its function.[12] If this happens while you're pregnant, it can lead to premature delivery, preeclampsia, and birth defects in the fetus. Hypothyroidism has been shown to have a negative effect on a mother's milk supply and infant weight gain if left untreated.[13]

Conversely, in rare cases, hypothyroidism can increase the levels of thyrotropin-releasing hormone (TRH). This hormone increases the production of prolactin and can lead to oversupply.[14] However, low milk supply is more often associated with hypothyroidism, and oversupply is rare.

Postpartum Thyroiditis

Hyperthyroidism, or an overactive thyroid, is an autoimmune condition marked by increased levels of the thyroid hormone thyroxine. High levels of thyroxine combined with low levels of thyroid-stimulating hormone (TSH) are typically indicative of hyperthyroidism. Like hypothyroidism, the symptoms of hyperthyroidism are similar to that of many other diseases, as well as some of the normal symptoms of the immediate postpartum period: fatigue, difficulty sleeping, thinning hair, changes in bowel patterns, increased metabolism (which leads to increased hunger and weight loss), nervousness, anxiousness, or irregular heartbeat.

Postpartum thyroiditis is a condition characterized by transient (temporary) hyperthyroidism that occurs in the first year postpartum and affects an estimated 5 to 10 percent of women in the United States.[15] Although genetic and environmental variances tend to affect the incidence of postpartum thyroiditis, scientists don't yet know what these factors are, because studies looking at women within the same country show a wide variation of incidence. It's believed that postpartum thyroiditis is also a manifestation of a subclinical autoimmune disease of the thyroid that existed prior to a woman's pregnancy and is exacerbated in the immediate postpartum period.[16] This suppression and then exacerbation of symptoms can be seen in most pregnant women with autoimmune diseases. Women will often report that their rheumatoid arthritis, Crohn's disease, or multiple sclerosis symptoms are improved during pregnancy only to flare immediately postpartum. Women with postpartum thyroiditis generally develop hyperthyroidism between two to six months postpartum, and this eventually changes to hypothyroidism within three to twelve months postpartum.[17] When thyroid function changes from hyperthyroidism to hypothyroidism, it sometimes results in permanent hypothyroidism. However, as is the mysterious nature of most autoimmune diseases, it doesn't always follow a predictable pattern. Some women only develop hyperthyroidism, and others only develop hypothyroidism. Unlike other forms of thyroid disease, postpartum thyroiditis can't be prevented with iodine intake in the diet or with iodine supplementation.

Postpartum thyroiditis can often go undiagnosed as most of the symptoms are synonymous with being a new mother. Symptoms include:[18]

Lack of energy
Irritability
Nervousness
Sweating
Dry skin
Shaking hands
Depression
Heat intolerance
Dry hair
Puffy face
Hair falling out
Weight loss
Constipation
Aches and pains
Cold intolerance
Poor memory
Lack of concentration

If you believe you may have a thyroid issue, talk to your physician about it right away.

PROLACTIN DEFICIENCY

Hypoprolactinemia, also known as prolactin deficiency, is a rare condition in which your body doesn't make enough prolactin. Infertility, subfertility, menstrual disorders, and delayed puberty have all been associated with prolactin deficiency.[19] Prolactin is such an important part of the body's ability to produce milk that even in the absence of a true deficiency, suboptimal prolactin levels can have a negative impact on breast milk production. In addition to hypoprolactinemia's effect on lactation, lower than normal levels of prolactin are associated with lower immune function.[20] Many of the lactogenic foods and galactagogues we will explore in this book enhance immune function in addition to increasing milk production.

INFERTILITY SECONDARY TO PITUITARY DISORDERS

Infertility can have many causes, from structural to hormonal. Sometimes there's only one factor affecting one's ability to conceive, and sometimes multiple factors, both structural and hormonal, are the cause. If you had infertility problems caused by a prolactin deficiency (which is typically due to a pituitary disorder), then there's an increased likelihood that you will not make enough prolactin to generate a sufficient amount of milk to feed your baby. If you're currently struggling with infertility but plan to breastfeed in the future, then it's a good idea to have your prolactin levels checked. Whether you become a parent through traditional conception, IUI, IVF, egg or sperm donation, surrogacy, or adoption, breastfeeding is still an option, and it's helpful to have these baseline prolactin levels available when evaluating your milk supply once your little one has arrived.

SHEEHAN'S SYNDROME

Sheehan's syndrome, also known as Simmonds' syndrome or postpartum hypopituitarism, is a condition marked by decreased functioning of the pituitary gland. This decrease in function is typically due to trauma at birth, such as hypovolemic shock or blood loss leading to tissue damage during and/or directly after childbirth. This trauma causes damage to the pituitary gland and has a ripple effect that decreases or halts the storage, production, and secretion of pituitary hormones. Because prolactin is made in the pituitary gland, Sheehan's syndrome has a direct, negative effect on lactation. Typically, the first sign that a mother might have Sheehan's syndrome is either the complete absence of the ability to produce breast milk or initial difficulties producing enough breast milk to nourish her child sufficiently. In addition to decreased prolactin production, Sheehan's syndrome can also cause a decrease in thyroid-stimulating hormone (TSH), cortisol, growth hormones, and gonadotropins (hormones that affect fertility). While postpartum hemorrhage is a common complication of pregnancy, Sheehan's syndrome is a rare complication of postpartum hemorrhage.[21]

HORMONAL BIRTH CONTROL

Exclusively breastfeeding is associated with temporary amenorrhea and decreased fertility for at least the first six months postpartum. *Amenorrhea* means the absence of a menstrual cycle including ovulation and menses. This phenomenon is known as lactation-induced amenorrhea, and using breastfeeding as a method of birth control is called the lactational amenorrhea method, or LAM. The LAM method is over 98 percent effective if used correctly for the initial six-month postpartum period.[22] However, just as there are strict protocols around the use of hormonal birth control methods, there are protocols around the use of LAM. In order for LAM to be effective, the following criteria must be met:

- The baby must be exclusively breastfeeding

- The infant must nurse directly at the breast for at least ten short or six long nursing sessions within a twenty-four-hour period

- Supplemental feedings (including expressed breast milk and formula) can be no more than 1 ounce (30 ml) per week in the first month, 2 ounces (60 ml) per week in the second month, and 3 ounces (90 ml) per week in the third month.

- There can be no replacement of direct breastfeeding with formula or expressed breast milk feedings, and no more than 10 percent of feedings or foods can be something other than breast milk.

- Breastfeeding must be maintained throughout the day and night with no long intervals between breastfeeding. (LAM is no longer effective if there's a single interval of ten hours without breastfeeding or more than two feedings that are six hours apart through the duration that the LAM method is used.)

For a variety of reasons, many new mothers in the United States choose not to use (or may have trouble sticking to) the LAM protocol and therefore turn to other forms of contraception. Nonhormonal methods such as condoms and nonhormonal IUDs (such as ParaGard) don't have any reported negative effects on breastfeeding, but hormonal birth control methods can, depending on the method chosen. In general, women who choose a hormonal method of birth control are encouraged to wait until breastfeeding is well established before initiating their preferred method.

There are currently over one hundred different types of birth control pills, patches, vaginal rings, IUDs, and implanted birth control methods available on the market in the United States—and everyone responds differently to each one. Some women, even when using a hormonal birth control method that hasn't been shown to have any negative effects on breastfeeding, will experience a decrease in milk supply once a hormonal birth control is initiated. However, some hormonal birth control methods have had proven negative effects on milk supply. Here is a breakdown of the hormonal methods we know about:

- Levonorgestrel IUDs (common brand names Mirena and Skyla) have been shown to decrease breastfeeding performance when inserted prior to six weeks postpartum but had little to no negative effect on breastfeeding when inserted past six weeks postpartum.[23]
- Progestogen-only injectables (common brand names Depo-Provera, Megestron, and Petogen) were shown to have little to no negative effect on breastfeeding when initiated before or after the six-week-postpartum period.[24] Findings were consistent when looking at etonogestrel implants (common brand names Nexplanon and Implanon).[25]
- Oral contraceptives that use a combination of the hormones estrogen and progestogen (the typical birth control pill) are usually best avoided if you want to maintain a healthy milk supply. There's inconclusive evidence about the use of the combination pill, but most studies have found some link between a

decline in breastfeeding and breast milk supply in women utilizing combined hormonal oral contraception.[26] If you're using the combination pill, wait as long as possible to go on it again after giving birth. The longer a mother waits to initiate use of a combined hormonal oral contraceptive method, the better her chances are to breastfeed successfully.

- Progestogen-only oral contraception, also known as the mini-pill, has the most favorable data in protecting and maintaining a woman's breast milk supply and quality. However, it's worth mentioning that an association has been found between using oral contraceptives and a moderate level of the hormone used in the contraceptive appearing in a woman's breast milk.[27]

If you're taking hormonal birth control and experience a decline in your milk volume, it can happen rapidly or slowly over time. Therefore, make sure to pay close attention to your infant's feeding cues (see page 17) and any changes in milk volume that might be present. If you believe your milk supply may have been negatively affected by hormonal birth control methods, talk to your doctor about finding the right birth control option for you while breastfeeding, and consider using a nonhormonal method while breastfeeding. If you're able to switch methods, lactogenic foods and herbs like the ones found in Chapter 9 can be incredibly effective tools in increasing your milk supply again.

INFANT ANATOMICAL ABNORMALITIES

Tongue- and Lip Ties

Tongue-ties and lip ties are two of the most common anatomical abnormalities that can negatively affect feeding in the short and long term. They can have a negative impact on not only breastfeeding but also feeding through early childhood and adulthood.

The technical term for a tongue-tie is *ankyloglossia*. It's part of a larger group of anatomical abnormalities that occur within the womb when the fetus is approximately eight weeks gestational age, far before most women know they are pregnant. A tongue-tie is characterized by an abnormal lingual frenulum—the thin membrane that connects the underside of the tongue to the bottom of the mouth—that limits tongue movement. While later in life the hallmark problem of a restrictive tongue is a lisp or other speech problems, in infants it can cause a variety of medical issues for both mother and baby. For your little one, a restrictive tongue-tie can cause high or bubble palate (due to the tongue's lack of mobility during formation of the oral cavity in utero), abnormal swallowing, abnormal weight gain, failure to thrive, reflux, problems with the introduction of solid foods, and upper and lower gastrointestinal distress.[28] A tongue-tie can also cause an infant to dislike nursing or any other forms of true suckling, as attempting to extend the tongue can prove to be painful. For breastfeeding mothers, an infant with a tongue-tie can cause nipple pain/soreness, nipple trauma (including cracks and bleeding), low milk supply, and recurrent plugged ducts (see page 40). If a restrictive tie isn't released, the long-term complications can include dental and orthodontic issues, gagging and choking on solid food, chewing difficulties, mouth breathing, facial esthetic changes, orofacial myofunctional disorders,

sleep apnea, and speech problems.[29]

While a tongue-tie restricts an infant's tongue mobility, an upper lip tie can negatively affect an infant's ability to create an effective seal for milk removal while suckling. To compensate for not being able to flange out her lips completely, an infant might tuck her lower lip in or overcompensate with the chin and jaw to create an effective seal, causing pain while nursing and, in some cases, damage to the nipple. Additionally, in the absence of a suitable lip seal, infants can take in too much air while nursing, which can result in reflux, upper and lower gastrointestinal pain, gassiness, and fussiness.[30]

Current data is inconsistent on the number of infants born with a tongue-tie. It's estimated that anywhere from 4 to 11 percent of newborns are born with a tongue-tie,[31] however, approximately 66 percent of infants whose mothers reach out to an outpatient clinic or lactation consultant because of breastfeeding difficulties have tongue-ties.[32] For this reason, if you're having breastfeeding issues, it's paramount that you make sure to find a provider well versed in tongue- and lip tie diagnosis and release.

Not all tongue-ties or lip ties are created equally. At times, a tie can appear restrictive but when function is observed, as in during a suck evaluation or nursing session, the infant is able to nurse efficiently and effectively at the breast. Other times a tie might be barely noticeable (these are often referred to as posterior tongue-ties), yet they have a negative impact on an infant's ability to transfer milk and can cause significant nipple pain to the breastfeeding mother. This is why it's always important to be evaluated by a health care professional who has been specifically educated on how to identify and evaluate a tongue- or lip tie properly.

Unfortunately, most pediatricians aren't trained on how to identify or treat tongue-ties and lip ties or understand their effect on breastfeeding. An International Board Certified Lactation Consultant is a great resource for identifying a tongue-tie, evaluating form and function, as well as giving advice on how to help an infant learn to suck properly with and without a surgical procedure. Other qualified health care professionals well versed in diagnosis and treatment of tongue-ties are pediatric dentists, orthodontists, and pediatric ear, nose, and throat (ENT) specialists. A speech language pathologist is also an invaluable member of the feeding team if tongue-tie is affecting an infant's ability to swallow or if an infant is having issues with aspiration. However, it should be noted that tongue- and lip ties tend to be a subspecialty, and not all IBCLCs, dentists, orthodontists, ENTs, and/or speech language pathologists are well versed in the identification, treatment, and aftercare of a tie.

Treatment for most major tongue- and lip ties is a release procedure called a frenotomy, in which the portion of the frenulum causing restriction is clipped with either a scalpel, scissors, or laser. Different providers use different techniques to release a tie, but one method isn't necessarily better than the next. Many pediatric ENTs prefer to use scissors, while pediatric dentists will often choose a laser, since it's used for a variety of in-office procedures and it's the tool they're most comfortable with.

No matter what method is used, it's effective: In one study, nearly 91 percent of breastfeeding mothers reported some degree of breastfeeding improvement after a frenotomy, while 100 percent of breastfeeding mothers reported some degree of breastfeeding improvement with release of an upper lip tie.[33] And in a systematic review of twelve studies on the effectiveness of a frenotomy, researchers found there were no major complications from the procedure.[34]

However, for many infants, the release of a tie in and of itself won't automatically correct all of their breastfeeding issues. Many infants will have to relearn how to suck with their new oral anatomy. No matter how old your infant is when her tongue-tie is released, she has had this anatomical structure her entire life, and it's all been changed in a day! This requires quite a bit of adjustment on your baby's part and patience and persistence on your part as the breastfeeding mother. Finding an IBCLC trained in teaching infants to suck after a frenotomy is equally as important as having the tie released. Some infants might require occupational therapy by a pediatric occupational therapist trained specifically in teaching an infant how to suck effectively at the breast. Additionally, case studies have shown that chiropractic care for your baby postfrenotomy provided by a chiropractor who specializes in pediatrics can be a helpful adjunct to the care of a breastfeeding infant.[35]

Cleft Lip or Cleft Palate

While tongue- and lip ties aren't always overtly obvious to the untrained eye, a cleft lip, cleft palate, or a combination of both is. This facial abnormality can even usually be spotted on an ultrasound while your child is in utero, giving you plenty of time to work with your health care team to come up with a proposed plan for feeding. No two clefts are the same, and, therefore, each case's plan of care will be different, although nursing at the breast is typically easier for a child who has a cleft lip with no palate involvement. Finding a lactation consultant who is experienced in working with children with anatomical abnormalities will help tremendously in positioning and latching a child with a cleft. For mothers who have an infant with a cleft lip or palate, and therefore an inefficient suck, it's typically necessary to either pump or hand express milk after a nursing session to ensure that your milk supply stays strong.

There is still so much research that needs to be done in regard to clefts and breastfeeding. However, the studies that we do have show what a marked difference cultural norms have on breastfeeding initiation rates and sustaining the breastfeeding relationship. In countries where breastfeeding is the societal norm, 100 percent of mothers initiated breastfeeding with infants who had cleft lips, cleft palates, or a combination of both.[36] On average, mothers were able to exclusively breastfeed for a little over two weeks before beginning to supplement with expressed breast milk or formula. Even more remarkable is that these mothers were able to initiate and sustain breastfeeding for this time period without consulting any outside lactation support or counseling. In the United States, where breastfeeding isn't the societal norm, initiation rates tend to be very low, and many mothers don't sustain exclusive breastfeeding for long.

BIRTHING METHODS AND MEDICATIONS GIVEN DURING BIRTH

Many mothers don't realize that medications used in labor, such as epidural anesthetic or Demerol, can affect the baby's ability to latch on and breastfeed effectively. Some studies show these effects last as long as a month, depending on the medication used in the epidural and the length of time the mother received it.

Certain birthing methods also carry more risks of causing nursing problems later. Of all the birthing methods presently studied, birthing via a cesarean section has the greatest association with breastfeeding difficulties and has a direct, negative impact on initiating and sustaining breastfeeding.[37] This birthing method is associated with delayed onset of lactogenesis[38] (see Chapter 3 for an explanation of the process of lactogenesis). This phenomenon is consistent among both elective and emergency cesarean sections; however, emergency C-sections are associated with lower levels of prolactin production than elective C-sections or vaginal delivery.[39] This is not to say that all mothers who give birth via C-section or use medical interventions such as an epidural anesthetic or Pitocin will have trouble breastfeeding. However, these procedures do increase the risk that breastfeeding will get off to a rocky start.

If you did have one of these procedures while giving birth or are pregnant and your birth plan includes them, it's important to look at this information as empowering rather than defeating. With this knowledge, you can better create a birthing and postpartum care plan for yourself and your baby that will optimize the breastfeeding relationship while acknowledging the difficulties that may arise and preparing for them. Above all else, it will be imperative to have your support system in place to help you and your baby manage the transition from birth to breastfeeding.

RETAINED PLACENTA

As I mentioned in Chapter 3, lactogenesis II (more commonly referred to as a mother's milk "coming in") is triggered by birth, but not the birth of the baby—the birth of the placenta. Once the placenta has fully detached and been delivered, a decline begins in the hormone progesterone, which helps maintain a healthy pregnancy. The sharp decline of progesterone in the presence of high levels of prolactin and cortisol signal the body to transition from lactogenesis I to lactogenesis II, and by day three to seven postpartum a mother will have transitioned from colostrum to mature milk.[40] If any part of the placenta isn't delivered, then the body will

still produce levels of progesterone that are too high to allow a full, mature milk supply to be present. If you have concerns about your milk supply that you believe might be due to a retained placenta, this is an excellent time to have your physician check to be sure the placenta was completely delivered. Your two- or six-week postpartum OB-GYN visit is a great time to do this.

PRETERM BIRTHS

I make no secret of the fact that premature babies are some of my favorite people on earth. While they might be small, they have no shortage of personality, making up for any shortcoming with spunk, toothless grins, and a long list of opinions they express in their actions and inactions. They know they might not be able to do all the things they want to do just yet, but they don't care! Unfortunately, one of the things they are often not able to do is effectively nurse. Your breasts start making milk early on in your pregnancy so that they're ready even if your baby comes early. This means that even if your baby comes earlier than expected, your body is ready with breast milk made specifically for your infant's needs. However, there are several factors that can inhibit the breastfeeding relationship between a mother and her premature baby. From tube feeds to increased separation due to time spent in the NICU, it can be a tough road, but, for many, a road that does lead to a vibrant breastfeeding relationship.

For infants born before thirty-two weeks, one of the primary challenges to the physical act of breastfeeding is that they have not yet developed the coordination necessary to suckle effectively at the breast. While you might have observed your little one sucking her fingers in the womb during an ultrasound, this suck isn't strong and effective enough to draw milk from the breast. For infants born past thirty-two weeks, a common physical barrier to breastfeeding is that their buccal fat pads and muscles haven't developed in their cheeks and jaws to the extent needed to create the suction necessary to nurse effectively at the breast.

If you aren't able to nurse immediately after the birth of your preemie, begin to hand express colostrum on a regular basis (eight to twelve times a day) until lactogenesis II begins at around one to three days postpartum (see pages 74–75 for tips on how to successfully hand express). Once this happens and you begin to make mature milk, use a hospital-grade pump every two to three hours to provide milk for your infant via an alternative feeding device such as a feeding syringe, finger feeder, or supplemental nursing system. Avoid early introduction of bottles to an infant who doesn't have the strength or coordination to properly suckle at the breast, as it typically causes problems with nipple aversion when trying to move the infant from bottle-feeding to breastfeeding.

OVERWEIGHT AND OBESITY

Excess body weight does more than increase your risk of developing type 2 diabetes, cardiovascular disease (including heart attack, stroke, and hypertension), and certain types of cancers. Research has now shown that being overweight (having a body mass index higher than 25) and, especially, being obese (having a BMI higher than 30) can have a direct effect on the production, storage, and use of a wide range of hormones. In breastfeeding mothers, one hormone that has been studied extensively in relation to excess body weight and obesity is prolactin.

Research has shown that the highest prevalence of undesired weaning is reported by obese mothers, followed by overweight mothers.[41] This is due, primarily, to a decrease in prolactin levels in mothers who are overweight or obese at the start of their pregnancy. It would seem that overweight and obese women have a lower prolactin response to suckling, meaning that, even when practicing on-demand nursing and with no other nursing problems present, overweight and obese mothers begin to make less prolactin starting at forty-eight hours postpartum and extending to the seventh day postpartum.[42] The timing of this drop in prolactin is crucial. As you'll recall from Chapter 3, this is a critical time in which lactogenesis I ends and lactogenesis II begins. Approximately 44 percent of obese women who are able to initiate and sustain breastfeeding have a delayed lactogenesis II, meaning that it can take significantly longer for their milk to transition from colostrum to mature milk.[43]

It's important to note that not all mothers who are overweight or obese at the time of conception will have breastfeeding difficulties or delayed lactogenesis. Just as I urged you to be empowered with knowledge rather than discouraged if your little one is born with an abnormality, I encourage you to not be hard on yourself if you're overweight or obese. Check out pages 93–95 for some guidance on how to safely lose weight postpartum, as well as Chapter 9 for information about herbs and lactogenic foods that work primarily by increasing prolactin levels. These can be a vital tool in helping to decrease the lag time between lactogenesis I and II.

NONMEDICAL REASONS FOR LOW MILK SUPPLY

The nonmedical reasons for low milk supply far exceed the medical reasons I discussed in the last chapter in scope and prevalence. And the good news is that, for the grand majority of women, they're entirely fixable. Although the medical conditions discussed in Chapter 5 are much rarer than the nonmedical causes of low milk supply covered in this chapter, it's important to treat them before you move on to other ways you can increase your breast milk. Make sure you take a look through the previous chapter and consult with a physician and/or lactation consultant for treatment if necessary.

Unfortunately, when it comes to breastfeeding, Western culture is full of more misinformation than good education and more myth than fact. More often than not, low milk supply is a man-made issue born of a century of falsehoods circulated about breastfeeding and breast milk and societal birthing and parenting norms. Since the 1930s, the majority of infants in the United States have been formula fed. Multiple generations of Western men and women have never seen breastfeeding and know very little about it beyond the adage "breast is best." We rely on our village of other parents to be our guides along our journey, and they don't always steer us in the right direction.

But what does this ultimately mean for you and your own breastfeeding journey? It means that, for the grand majority of women, milk supply issues are preventable and fixable.

As you start to read through this chapter you might find yourself tempted to blame yourself for your low milk supply. This chapter is here as a tool of empowerment not of blame or guilt. As parents, and as people, we do the very best we can for our children and ourselves with the information we have. You aren't expected to be perfect or to know it all. Use this chapter to prevent breastfeeding issues before they begin, but if you're already having trouble breastfeeding or think you have a low milk supply, don't panic. Instead, reach out to an International Board Certified Lactation Consultant, or another parent you trust. Seeking support at the first sign of breastfeeding troubles is key to helping you uncover the reason(s) behind low milk supply and fixing it.

INEFFECTIVE SUCK OR LATCH

If you haven't taken a look at the section on figuring out if your baby is getting enough milk (pages 35–38), go back and make sure that your baby is latching and sucking effectively. Signs that he has an ineffective suck or latch are if he has slow weight gain and/or low urine and stool output, and if you have pain when nursing, nipple soreness, or any nipple trauma, or if your nipple shape changes immediately following a nursing session.

There are a variety of causes for an ineffective latch or suck, and many—like preterm delivery, infant anatomical abnormalities, or a traumatic birth—are relatively unavoidable. But one major cause of an infant not being able to latch or suck well enough is 100 preventable: the early introduction of bottles and pacifiers.

Bottle-feeding is still the societal norm in the United States. Because of this, many infants receive bottles before breastfeeding is well established. Though some mothers have no choice but to be separated from their babies and rely on bottle feedings, oftentimes bottle-feeding is presented as an opportunity to give a mother who is currently at home a "break" from the task of infant feeding, to allow the mother's partner a chance to bond with the baby through feeding, or to ensure that the baby will take a bottle later. These reasons all have the potential to negatively affect a woman's milk supply. The sentiments of friends and family members who want to give a new mother a break from infant feeding are kind and appreciated, but they do not support a long-term breastfeeding relationship between mother and baby. Try as we might, we can't fool our bodies into continually making milk that will exclusively support the nursing needs of an infant if we aren't breastfeeding exclusively. Any time a mother is separated from her baby, she must pump or hand express milk—there's no way around this. So (whether they like it or not) mothers never truly get a break from infant feeding—they still must stop, pump, and then clean the pump's parts and bottles. In the time that takes, she could have nursed her child and maybe even had a couple of extra minutes to spare. That's why I always encourage mothers who are available to nurse to do so, instead of pumping.

The best way to support a breastfeeding mother and truly give her a break is to help take all other duties except infant feeding off of her plate for as long as possible. The common advice to "sleep when the baby sleeps" is nearly an impossible one. If every parent slept when their infant slept, there would be no time to eat, put a load of laundry in the washing machine, clean the dishes, shower, or at the very least change into a new set of pajamas. However, if all a mother has to do is nurse, and she can worry as little as possible about who's going to cook dinner, or unload the dishwasher, or even change the baby's diaper, then she can truly focus on resting and building the foundations of strong breastfeeding skills in her infant.

Especially during the first year of a baby's life, it can feel to parents like the burden of parenthood falls more squarely on the shoulders of the breastfeeding mother. But even if it may feel like the breastfeeding mother is doing all of the heavy lifting of parenting, a good partner does much more than simply play a supporting role. It's extremely difficult for a mother to sustain a healthy breastfeeding relationship with her infant if she doesn't have a strong support system surrounding her, and for many women, the main source of support in their homes is their partner. However, it's important for partners to remember that their job is still support, and not the feeding itself.

We have come a long way from dads anxiously sitting in the waiting room waiting to be told their child is born—now partners aren't only in the delivery room but jumping in the birthing tub during labor, providing counterpressure through contractions, and being steady and confident coaches throughout labor and delivery. Once their little ones are born, many partners want to continue that involvement in any way they can, and infant feeding seems like the next logical step in not only care but bonding. However, feeding in and of itself isn't bonding. Remember all the things you learned about oxytocin in Chapter 3? The all-important love hormone that's released every time a mother nurses, oxytocin is nature's way of ensuring that the bond between mother and baby is strengthened with every feeding. But when an infant bottle-feeds, there's no rush of oxytocin bonding the person holding the bottle to the baby. There's simply feeding. In the long list of tasks that are required of a parent in a twenty-four-hour period, feeding via a bottle is probably the most passive of them all. If your partner is looking for a way to bond with your baby, ditch the bottle and try these options instead:

Holding skin-to-skin
Rocking
Soothing
Burping
Dancing
Playing
Diapering
Bathing
Massaging
Cuddling
Laughing

This is a time to think of your little one as a tiny human. When we humans are upset, we want someone to comfort us, to provide a loving hug, a listening ear. When we're feeling playful, we want someone to laugh at our jokes and funny faces. When we're tired, we want someone to be a soothing presence to help us transition into slumber. When a non-breastfeeding parent provides love and care through soothing, singing, laughing, dancing, and even diaper changes, those are the moments that bond them to their baby. Yes, Mother Nature gave moms a hormonal running head start with oxytocin, but there are so many things a partner can do to catch up that don't involve feeding and that, in the end, will help strengthen the breastfeeding relationship even more.

NIPPLE SHIELDS

Nursing shields are a thin piece of silicone in the shape of an exaggerated nipple, placed over the mother's nipple to facilitate nursing. It has always been difficult for me to understand, as an outpatient lactation consultant, why nipple shields would be handed out so freely at the hospital level, as I see them cause a great deal of issues once a mother and baby are discharged. Discussion with hospital lactation consultants over the years has shown the answer comes down to time constraints and confidence. In the hospital setting, even though a lactation consultant might have a few hours with each patient, it is the first and only time she sees the mother and baby, so there is pressure to fix all nursing issues at that time. Nipple shields provide a quick way to help an infant latch and to reduce sore nipples and, when used properly, can be the bridge that connects mother to baby. When mothers are instructed on the proper way to use a nipple shield, with a thorough care plan, infants can gain weight well with the short-term use of a silicone nipple shield.[1] However, it is still a Band-Aid over the underlying cause of the nursing problem and can often create new nursing problems.

Just like bottles, many babies can get hooked on the nursing shield from the very first use. Nipple shields, like bottles, are designed to have long nipples that automatically touch an infant's hard palate when put in the mouth, stimulating the sucking reflex. When a mom nurses using the bare nipple, it is the job of the infant to open his mouth wide and take in enough of the areola and nipple to touch the hard palate and stimulate the sucking reflex. Essentially, nursing means that an infant must actively suck and work to eat, while a nursing shield does not encourage an infant to have a good, wide latch in order to stimulate sucking.

Mothers with a robust milk supply or oversupply typically have the best success with a nipple shield in the long term, as the lower milk transfer caused by the nipple shield does not tend to adversely affect the amount of milk their infant receives. However, mothers who are already struggling with low milk supply or have a normal milk supply often find that nursing with a nipple shield inhibits the amount of milk that their infant can transfer at each nursing session, leading to slower weight gain and a further decrease in milk supply. Additionally, due to decreased milk transfer with the use of a nipple shield, a mother's risk of developing plugged ducts, mastitis, and thrush increases.[2]

For all these reasons, it is important to not just put a Band-Aid over your infant's nursing problems with a nipple shield but work with a lactation consultant to get to the bottom of those problems and find a solution that works best for your family.

SUPPLEMENTING WITH FORMULA

I've discussed some reasons for not using formula throughout this book, perhaps the greatest being that the more your baby is away from your breast, the less milk you will make. But feeding your baby formula does more than just interfere with your body's natural responses to nursing. Formula changes the entire way your baby eats. It's not easy to digest, and, in fact, very few of the synthetic vitamins and minerals in formula are readily absorbed by the body. While easy-to-digest breast milk takes about an hour and a half to be digested, formula takes approximately four hours. This longer digestion time makes formula rougher on your baby's sensitive and immature gastrointestinal (GI)

tract, causing irritation and inflammation of the gut.

In 1991, the Baby-Friendly Hospital Initiative (BFHI) was developed by the World Health Organization and UNICEF to set up guidelines to help mothers and babies get off to the strongest start possible with breastfeeding in the hospital or birth center setting. The process of becoming a certified Baby-Friendly facility takes thousands of hours of provider and staff training and education as well as a demonstrated commitment to the care and support of breastfeeding mothers and babies. Baby-Friendly facilities aren't permitted to accept gifts from formula companies or provide formula company–sponsored gift bags filled with free formula to mothers. Ideally, in Baby-Friendly hospitals and birthing centers, formula is only used where medically indicated. With the increasing implementation of the BFHI around the United States, the inappropriate use of formula is decreasing, but we still have a long way to go.

The guidelines and recommendations for supplementing breast milk with formula that I list below are based on the most up-to-date (by the time of publication) clinical research on infant nutrition and medical nutrition therapy as it pertains to expressed breast milk, donor milk, fortified milk, and formula supplementation.

When Is It Medically Necessary to Supplement Breast Milk?

The Academy of Breastfeeding Medicine's protocol on supplementary feedings for healthy infants is the gold standard in evidence-based information on medical nutrition therapy via breast milk or formula for newborn infants. These are the standards by which all other major infant-feeding protocols are based, including those used in certified Baby-Friendly hospitals. They state that the only times you should supplement breastfeeding with bottle-feeding for a full-term, healthy infant are when:[3]

1. There is a separation due to maternal illness such as shock, sepsis, or psychosis, and/or if mother and baby are at two separate hospitals.

2. The infant is born with an inborn error of metabolism such as galactosemia or PKU.

3. The infant is unable to feed at the breast due to medical reasons

such as congenital malformation or illness.

4. The mother is taking medications that are contraindicated with breastfeeding.

Additionally, supplementation may be necessary if the mother has a medical reason for low milk supply, such as delayed lactogenesis II due to a retained placenta, Sheehan's syndrome, primary glandular insufficiency, or prior breast surgery.[4] (See Chapter 5 for more on these conditions.)

These protocols clearly state that the first choice for supplementation is expressed human milk; the second choice, if available, is prescreened, pasteurized donor milk; and the third choice is protein hydrolysate formula, also known as elemental formula. Elemental formulas are preferred over standard formulas to ensure that the infant isn't exposed to the protein in cow's milk (beta-casein).

When Is It Unnecessary to Supplement?

Many times bottle-feeding and formula supplementation is presented in the hospital setting as being a medically necessary intervention when it's not. Unfortunately, the problem is compounded when the medical information being given isn't based on the current scientific evidence or guidelines, but on old advice that's been passed down from one health care provider to another. If your health care provider suggests the use of formula in the following circumstances, you should be aware that they may not be based on the current guidelines.

GREATER THAN 10 PERCENT WEIGHT LOSS

Infant weight loss, and more specifically the percentage of weight loss after birth, is one of the principal measures that hospital and outpatient pediatricians use to determine if an infant is transferring colostrum well and getting the hydration and nutrients necessary for growth and development. But as I discussed on page 37, the guidelines that many doctors use for after-birth weight loss are 4 to 7 percent, which is based solely on the growth pattern of formula-fed infants.[5] Newer research suggests that 10 percent should be the maximum amount of weight loss considered normal in breastfed infants. If an infant has lost more than 10 percent of his

initial body weight, the health care provider will most likely begin evaluating him for breastfeeding issues, typically recommending that the mother begin supplementing her infant's diet with formula.

Recent studies have shown, however, that a weigh loss of greater than 10 percent isn't a cause for alarm in all situations. Higher birth weight, female sex, cesarean section, epidural use, and a longer hospital stay have all been associated with greater infant weight loss in the hospital.[6] IV fluids during labor have also been shown to transfer to the baby and cause him to have a higher weight. In cases in which weight loss in the infant is primarily due to fluid loss, an increase in urine output within the first twenty-four hours of life is expected.[7] Because of this, it's recommended that if a mother receives IV fluids within two hours of birth, the infant's dry weight (weight after fluid loss) be taken twenty-four hours after birth, and this weight should be the reference point for weight loss.

It's also important to keep in mind that infant weight loss is just one data point to look at when evaluating effective feeding. Counting the number of wet and poopy diapers in a twenty-four-hour time period is another tool that should be used in conjunction with infant weight to evaluate breastfeeding in the first weeks of life (see pages 36–37 for more information on how to do this).

NEONATAL JAUNDICE

Jaundice is so common among babies that approximately 70 to 84 percent of full-term infants and over 80 percent of preterm infants will develop it.[8] Neonatal jaundice occurs when an infant's body contains too much bilirubin, a yellowish substance formed in the liver by the breakdown of hemoglobin in red blood cells. A natural antioxidant, bilirubin is present in everyone's blood and stool.[9] (In fact, bilirubin is what gives stool its characteristic brown color.) Jaundice, a yellowing in the skin caused by bilirubin, is considered the physiologic norm for most newborns, but if their bilirubin levels are too high, treatment may be initiated. Bilirubin lab values below 19 mg/dL are considered within the normal range, although the closer bilirubin levels creep toward 20, the more likely a pediatrician will order that an infant be put under bili-lights (phototherapy) to help him break down and eliminate excess bilirubin in the body. In general, clinical guidelines state that if, upon rechecking, the baby's bilirubin levels are decreasing, no treatment is typically needed as long as the infant is eliminating waste effectively.

Bilirubin levels tend to decrease more slowly in breastfed babies versus formula-fed babies; however, as long as bilirubin levels are steadily decreasing under the care of trained medical professionals, the risk of hyperbilirubinemia (dangerously high bilirubin levels) in jaundiced babies is low.[10] Colostrum—that nutrient-rich milk that your breasts produce right after giving birth—is a natural laxative that helps your baby eliminate any retained bilirubin through his stool.[11] In this case, your body works in harmony with your infant's to help bring bilirubin levels down to a normal level.

Phototherapy is the first-line treatment for infants with hyperbilirubinemia. Recent evidence suggest that infants can be removed from phototherapy for thirty minutes every three hours to breastfeed as needed, with some evidence showing that extended nursing breaks up to sixty minutes were beneficial to infants.[12] Additionally, breastfeeding mothers can request to sit under phototherapy with their little ones to allow for uninterrupted skin-to-skin contact as well as opportunity for nursing on demand.

Infants with jaundice tend to be sleepier and harder to wake for feedings. It can be tempting to let your baby sleep through a nursing session; however, for all infants, and especially for those with jaundice, it's paramount that your newborn be nursed at least eight to twelve times a day. Nursing within the first hour of life increases the odds that your baby will be able to successfully breastfeed in the immediate postpartum period. If an infant isn't nursed often and effectively in the first few days of his life, his risk of developing hyperbilirubinemia increases and his mother's milk supply decreases, which can mean a delay in lactogenesis II and suboptimal milk supply going forward. So make sure to feed your newborn at least every one to three hours, and offer him the breast often to encourage him to actively suck.

If an infant with jaundice is experiencing poor milk transfer that leads to bilirubin levels greater than 20 to 25 mg/dL, at the discretion of the health care provider, supplementation of breastfeeding may be necessary. If this is what your doctor recommends for your baby, you should know that supplementation with the mother's own milk via alternative feeding methods (referenced on page 6) is the first choice in current guidelines, followed by pasteurized donor milk, and lastly hydrolyzed protein (elemental) formulas. Elemental formulas have been shown to be more effective than standard formulas in preventing absorption of bilirubin and, therefore, enhancing excretion of bilirubin through the stool.[13] In most cases, only a small amount of elemental formula supplementation is needed to decrease bilirubin levels.

Lastly, while some health care providers might encourage the use of formula for treatment of jaundice in infants with bilirubin levels under 20 mg/dL, there's no clinical evidence to support this practice.

ENCOURAGING BABY TO SLEEP LONGER

Many times, in an effort to offer helpful advice to a new parent, a friend or family member might suggest using formula to help your little one sleep longer at night. While this can be a tempting option, it is also a good moment to take a step back and consider the reasons why an infant wakes up so often throughout the day and night. Infancy is a period of the most rapid physical and developmental growth your little one will ever experience. This accelerated rate of growth requires a great deal of calories and nutrients as well as sleep. Infants are typically pros at sleeping—getting upwards of twenty hours a day of sleep broken up into two- to four-hour segments throughout the day and night.

In the first few months of life, infants typically wake only to eat. Some infants will wake for a diaper change, but, with the new super-absorbent diapers, many infants do not even feel wet and will continue to sleep straight through a soiled diaper. As your little one gets older, eating will not be the only thing on his mind. He will be interested in exploring his world and learning about everything he can touch, taste, see, and smell, so his sleeping patterns may change as his eyesight and mobility improve.

Because breast milk is typically digested at a rate of approximately one and a half hours per feeding, an infant can be hungry anywhere from one to three hours after the start of his last feeding, and he will wake up to eat, even in the middle of the night. Your infant does not know day from night, and even if he did, he wouldn't care; the need to eat, grow, and thrive in a healthy way trumps the need to understand why the sun is up during the day and the moon lights the night! Because formula takes about three hours longer for an infant to digest, an infant will have the feeling of fullness for longer and take longer breaks between eating. This means that instead of waking anywhere from one to three hours after a feed, an infant might only wake every four to six hours. While it is true that an infant will sleep longer if he has had formula, the extra one to three hours of consecutive sleep come at the price of the baby's short-term and long-term nutritional needs.

REDUCING OR ELIMINATING NIGHTTIME FEEDINGS

The paradox of parenthood is that babies always seem to be asleep, yet parents are constantly tired. The moment your little baby bump began to show, everyone you know probably told you to get your rest now, because soon, sleep will be a distant memory of a thing you did once upon a time. Lack of sleep is the near-constant topic of parenting magazines, baby books, and every single conversation with new parents you will ever meet. But even though you know you're going to be tired, it's hard to conceptualize what that actually means until you're living it. When you're running off of thirty to forty-five minutes of sleep a day all while trying to do laundry, pay bills, cook dinner, and maybe even get in your first shower of the week, it's a good thing that the tiny little person you're taking care of— who is of no help in any of these categories—makes up for it in cuteness.

Meanwhile, especially with such little sleep, it can start to feel like something must be wrong with your baby. Is eating and sleeping all this sweet little person is supposed to do? And has no one told him that the moon rising means it's time for him (and his parents!) to get some sleep? But infants have two very basic needs besides love—food and sleep. From zero to eighteen months, your little one is experiencing the most rapid growth in his entire life, as you can probably tell from looking back on photos of him from only a month ago (he looks like a totally different person, doesn't he?). This rapid growth requires a lot of nutrients and energy (in the form of breast milk) and lots of sleep—twenty hours or more each day!

Why Nighttime Breastfeeding Is So Beneficial

During a twenty-four-hour cycle, your breast milk is constantly changing, as are the hormones that mediate its creation, storage, and removal. In particular, prolactin levels tend to be at their highest level in breastfeeding mothers at night.[14] This pattern follows our natural circadian rhythms that regulate our awake/sleep cycle. Reducing and/or eliminating nighttime feedings before an infant is ready to do so on his own disrupts this important cycle and tells your body to dramatically slow down its ability to make milk on a hormonal level.

Reducing or eliminating nighttime feedings not only has a negative impact on your supply, it reduces the amount of nutrients your child is able to take in and absorb in a day. The American Academy of Pediatrics launched a formal investigation into sleep-training techniques like Babywise to determine the extent of these types of sleep schedules on infant health. It found that infant feeding programs that eliminate or reduce nighttime feedings are linked to dehydration, failure to thrive, reduced milk supply, and involuntary early weaning.[15]

Getting Your Baby to Sleep

Newborns have immature senses, immune systems, and central nervous systems. They are unable to regulate body temperature and have very poor hormonal regulation, as well as poor eyesight. It takes months, years, and even decades for many of these systems to completely mature. An infant isn't born with a circadian rhythm. In fact, the circadian rhythm in infants doesn't begin to emerge developmentally until approximately ten to twelve weeks of age.[16]

The most important thing you can do to help your child have a peaceful night's sleep is to develop a nighttime routine. Routines are very different than schedules. A routine is simply the rituals that you and baby do every single day, no matter where you are. It helps signal that the end of the day is drawing near and provides a stable base for children to feel comfortable and secure before bedtime. For many, a bedtime routine consists of quieting the home environment, dimming the lights, giving your child

a bath or gentle massage, putting on pajamas, reading a bedtime story, and feeding. This routine evolves over time based on what is developmentally appropriate for an infant or child. Creating a solid and predictable routine will serve you much better in the long term than reducing or eliminating nighttime feedings in the short term—even if you don't remember the last time you stayed awake through a whole movie.

SCHEDULING FEEDINGS

Breastfeeding is the biological norm for all mammals, including humans. However, most industrialized nations have very low rates of breastfeeding. In the United States, breastfeeding fell out of favor as the social norm for feeding infants after the early 1900s, meaning that for many if not most American families, multiple generations haven't nursed for almost a hundred years. Due to this long period when breastfeeding simply wasn't socially favorable, most people weren't taught about the normal feeding and sleep patterns for an infant.

The typical guidelines for a breastfed infant are to nurse at least eight to twelve times a day. This rounds out to about every two to three hours (however, this can vary widely depending on the baby). Infants only know when they are uncomfortable or upset, and being hungry makes them feel both sensations at once. In developing countries where breast-feeding is the cultural norm, infants nurse an average of twelve to twenty times a day versus just five to six times a day in the United States.[17] In countries where breastfeeding is the cultural norm, mothers watch their babies and not the clock. They allow their infants to nurse on demand. Some nursing sessions are sixty minutes and some are five minutes. There's a very wide range of normal when it comes to how often an infant eats throughout the day and how long he nurses, and it's constantly evolving and changing as he changes and grows.

If you're evaluating whether you want your baby to be on a specific parent-imposed feeding schedule, take a step back and think of infants as what they are: tiny humans. In thinking of the eating patterns of adults, they are also highly variable. Sometimes you eat a satisfying lunch with all the carbohydrates, fat, and protein you need in the perfect proportions, but somehow an hour later you're hungry again. Sometimes you're hungry but sit down to eat and get distracted, or you get a headache or start to feel tired, so you decide to just take a few bites and come back and finish eating later. Sometimes you eat a small meal and feel satisfied for three to four hours. There is so much variation in how we eat and experience food daily. Infants have the exact same variation. This is why I advocate paying careful attention to an infant's cues. Breastfeeding on demand helps keep a mother's milk supply high and keeps baby full.

PACIFIER USE BETWEEN FEEDINGS

Infants suck in a very different manner than adults. In order to draw milk from the breast effectively, the tongue must pass the gum line. Try sucking your thumb with your tongue sticking out. It's a lot of work, isn't it? That hard work is designed to build the strength in an infant's head, neck, and jaw not only to suckle effectively now, but to speak, chew, and have proper oral development later. In order for an infant to suck on a pacifier, however, he has to push the pacifier up toward the roof of his mouth with his tongue to hold it in place. This is the opposite of what a good productive suck should look like. That's why it's no surprise that, introduced too soon, a pacifier can create poor sucking habits in infants, especially those who have underlying anatomical issues like those on pages 50–54. Until your infant has a strong grasp of proper tongue mobility, try not to use a pacifier.

Once nursing is well established, however, pacifiers can be a useful tool to help soothe your baby when it isn't possible for you to soothe him yourself, such as when you're traveling by car and can't immediately pick up or reach your little one to comfort him. Try to keep pacifier use to these kinds of emergency situations only, and don't just let it rest in his mouth between feedings or while he sleeps. Use Soothie-type pacifiers that have a cylindrical nipple and not flat-tip or orthodontic-tip pacifiers, which don't encourage the maintenance of a strong, productive suck.

In addition to harming your baby's suck, pacifiers can interfere with his feeding schedule. Many early signs of hunger involve babies' mouths, including rooting and putting their hands in their mouths. Some infants will even search for the breast with mouth open in nursing position as one of the final signs of hunger right before crying. Crying is a late sign of hunger—it's a sign that the baby has gone too long between feedings and is beyond the point of asking nicely. When an infant has a pacifier in his mouth between feedings, nearly all his early feeding cues can be missed. Additionally, infants who have a greater need to suck might continue to suck well beyond the point of hunger, only to finally express extreme hunger via high-pitched cries hours after the point they would have shown hunger in other ways, had they not been soothed by a pacifier. Because infants can go for longer stretches without nursing when pacifiers are used between feedings, this means they'll also likely nurse less often in a day, and, in response, a mother's milk supply may begin to dwindle.

INEFFECTIVE MILK EXPRESSION

For many mothers, having a reliable way to express milk is paramount. Some are separated from their little ones due to work, school, or other obligations. Other mothers may exclusively pump for premature or sick infants who can't suck.

There are a variety of ways to express milk from the breast. Manual and electric breast pumps are the preferred method for many mothers; however, breast pumps are actually a relatively new technology that has only been available commercially since the midnineties. Prior to this, the primary form of milk expression was hand expression. Hand expression tends to mimic breastfeeding better than pumping and can produce a higher yield of milk at each expression session. The method you choose to express milk when you're separated from your baby is up to you, as long as you're effectively removing as much milk as possible from the breast at each expression session (otherwise, your milk supply will begin to decrease). To learn how to evaluate your supply, see pages 33–38.

Choosing the Right Pump

A hospital-grade pump should be used if you're exclusively pumping for your baby. Hospital-grade pumps are the most durable of all pumps currently available on the market. They are composed of a closed system, meaning that no breast milk can enter the motor or other components of the pump. Due to this closed system, hospital-grade pumps can be used by multiple women. However, purchasing a hospital-grade pump is incredibly expensive, typically $1,500 to $2,000. Many women choose to rent a hospital-grade pump from a hospital or local reseller rather than purchasing, which can be a much more economical option.

Double-electric pumps are designed to be used by the mother who will only be separated from her infant for three to four nursing sessions a day, sometimes more. A double-electric pump is a great option for mothers who work outside the home, as they are typically much smaller, lighter, and easier to transport than hospital-grade pumps. Double-electric pumps usually have car chargers available as well, allowing moms to pump on the go. However, most double-electric pumps are open-system pumps, which means that there's a chance that small traces of milk can find their way into the motor. This poses a very small risk to a healthy full-term infant but can be detrimental to an immune-compromised infant. Additionally, because of this open system, it isn't recommended that double-electric breast pumps be shared mother to mother. A used double-electric pump, even if given by a close friend, isn't recommended. This is due not only to the open system of most pumps but also to the fact that commercial double-electric pump motors are built to typically last about one year, and the quality of suction can decline over time.

Manual pumps are a useful tool for the mother who will only occasionally be separated from her infant. For many mothers, expressions with a manual pump can take longer than with an electric pump, but with practice output typically improves. Manual pumps are lightweight and can fit easily into a glove compartment or purse. For this reason, I recommend that all moms who plan to be separated from their baby at any time have a manual pump around just in case. You never know when you will be without a good source of electricity or forget one of the many tubes and parts that go with an electric pump.

The vacuum pull from a pump might not always be effective for a variety of reasons, especially when it isn't working effectively or there's a gap somewhere in the tabs, flanges, or tubing that allows air to escape and thus decreases the vacuum pressure needed to pump effectively. A lactation consultant can use a specially designed pressure gauge to test if your breast pump is performing optimally.

Hand Expression

Hand expression is a method of milk expression that's closest to that of a baby's suckle. You don't have to worry about pump parts, access to a source of electricity, or anything more than a little soap and water to wash your hands prior to expression. Even if you plan on using a pump exclusively, it's always nice to learn how to hand express effectively in case you leave a part at home and can't pump or you find yourself unexpectedly without your pump. Trying to hand express properly under stress and pressure is difficult, so learning this skill when you're at home and relaxed is ideal.

When learning to hand express, there are two things you must never do—never squeeze the breast or pull out the nipple. This can cause internal and external bruising as well as tissue damage. Instead, you want to position your thumb at the top of your areola and two fingers underneath to support the areola from the underside. Gently push straight back into the chest wall without spreading your fingers and then roll your fingers and areola forward. Continue to repeat until milk ejection occurs and your breast is emptied. You can rotate your fingers around the areola to provide different pressure points for expression.

Getting the Most Out of Your Pump

Some women respond well to using a pump for milk expression, but the vacuum pull of a breast pump is very different than that of the rhythmic massage of an infant nursing. This mechanical difference typically means that a mother will pump less milk than she is actually producing. In my own practice, it isn't uncommon for a mother to come in with a concern about a pumping output of one to two ounces total only to reveal that her baby is transferring four ounces from one breast in a nursing session (see page 34 for more on why you shouldn't judge your output simply by what you pump).

When an infant is sucking effectively, there's no better way to remove milk from the breast. For this reason (and the many I gave in this chapter), I advise that you nurse rather than provide a bottle anytime you're with your baby. However, separation from your baby is often unavoidable, and some form of pumping is usually inevitable.

To maximize the amount of milk you get out of your pumping sessions, use a technique called Massage-Stroke-Shake, or MSS. MSS combines the gentle massaging of breastfeeding and hand expression with the vacuum seal created by a breast pump. This technique feels and looks a bit silly, but it's effective at stimulating oxytocin release, which increases the effectiveness of your letdowns when pumping or hand expressing.

Start by gently massaging your breasts, one a time, beginning at the chest wall and working in a circular motion until you reach the areola. This will look and feel similar to a breast self-examination (which, by the way, should be done monthly for all women over twenty years of age). After massaging, stroke from the top of the breast to the nipple with light tickle-like pressure. Continue around your breast until you have stroked the entire breast. Finally, lean forward and shake your breast for about ten to thirty seconds. You can do this prior to a pumping session or during a pumping session. Wearing a hands-free pumping bustier makes it easy to do the MSS technique while the pump is running to increase output even more.

Remember, nursing after a separation from your baby is paramount to helping protect your milk supply! If possible, get right back into breastfeeding as soon as you can after using a pump.

EARLY INTRODUCTION OF SOLID FOOD

The American Academy of Pediatrics (AAP), World Health Organization (WHO), Academy of Nutrition and Dietetics, and American Academy of Family Physicians (AAFP) all have guidelines and recommendations in place based on decades of research in pediatric nutrition and development that state emphatically that infants should be exclusively breastfed until at least six months of age. Exclusively breastfeeding means no formula (not even one bottle), solid foods, or any substance other than breast milk or necessary medications. All the scientific evidence currently available shows the greatest health advantages to children and adults who were exclusively breastfed for at least the first six months of life.

Despite these published guidelines, recommendations, and position papers, many pediatricians still erroneously advise parents to introduce solid foods at four months of age—sometimes even suggesting that a parent should introduce rice cereal mixed with expressed breast milk or formula in a bottle with a modified nipple earlier than four months. Not only are health care practitioners routinely recommending solid food introduction too soon, but many parents, in an effort to ensure their infant is getting the proper nutrition, introduce nonmilk liquids or solids too soon. One study of low-income mothers found that over a third of women introduced nonmilk liquids or solids seven to ten days postpartum. This number jumped up to 77 percent by eight weeks of age and 93 percent by sixteen weeks of age.[18]

Early introduction of solid foods often follows the belief that an infant doesn't appear satisfied after a feeding, seems ready to eat solid foods, or will sleep better at night.[19] When solid foods are introduced too early, it is often because caregivers do not know or understand the current guidelines for breastfeeding and solid food introduction or because they are worried about the quantity or quality of their breast milk.[20] If that's you, make sure to read pages 33–38, which cover evaluating your milk supply and whether or not your baby is getting enough nutrients with each feeding. If your baby appears hungry after a feeding, it might be because he's experiencing a growth spurt and is simply drinking more milk (see page 36), or he could have an ineffective latch or suck that's inhibiting the amount of milk that can be transferred in one nursing session (see page 59). Instead of turning to food supplementation for problems like these, it's important that you seek help with breastfeeding, preferably from an International Board Certified Lactation Consultant. You should also consult with a registered dietitian before changing the diet of an infant under six months old. And in case I got you excited with that mention of sleeping better at night, there's currently no clinical evidence that the early introduction of solid foods facilitates longer nighttime sleeping habits in infants.

You'll know your infant is developmentally ready to start solid foods when he can sit straight up 100 percent independently and accurately grab food, put it in his mouth, chew it, and swallow it. This rarely happens before six months of age without some type of assistance—don't rush it. When solid foods are introduced before six months of age, they're most likely going to replace a breastfeeding session. The less you nurse, the less milk you will make. I've had many mothers call my office in distress about a sharp decline in milk volume after introducing solids to their little ones a week or so prior!

Not only does introducing solid food too early lead to milk declines, solid foods aren't that beneficial for infants. As the saying goes, "Food before one is just for fun"—any food introduced between six months and a year shouldn't be meant to replace breast milk (or even formula) in your infant's diet but, instead, be a complement to it. Babies don't have the developmental capacity to eat and digest a nutrient-rich, balanced meal, which consists of a protein (legumes/beans, nuts/seeds, or meats), a starchy vegetable or grain, and vegetables and/or fruit. For them, breast milk is the perfect food containing all the vitamins, minerals, fat, carbohydrates, and protein they need at each meal. Not only that, but pureed foods are often heavily fruit based—even the vegetable blends that are currently available on the market have fruit and fruit juice as their primary ingredients. And while fruits are a healthy source of nutrients, they aren't appropriate in puree form due to the high sugar and low fiber content. So, 85 percent of an infant's diet should be breast milk until at least one year of age. Complementary foods should be added by baby-led introduction, which should significantly decrease the chances of a rapid decline in breastfeeding or breast milk production.[21] Letting your child lead the way means that you'll make just the right amount of breast milk that he needs for optimal nutrition while he experiments with solid food introduction.

MILK SLUMPS

Somewhere along your journey as a nursing mother, you will question your milk supply. It can seem as if you have finally gotten into a groove with nursing, and then suddenly your infant's behavior changes—she's nursing more often, nursing at both breasts when she only used to nurse on one side, or appearing to be on a nursing strike. If you're expressing milk to provide for your little one in bottles, you might notice that your pumping output has decreased dramatically overnight. Oftentimes these milk slumps (like those due to growth spurts or the return of your period) aren't permanent, and if you know they're coming, you can plan for them.

GROWTH SPURTS

An infant's first year of life is a time of rapid growth. Not even the dramatic growth spurts of the teen years can compare with the unprecedented growth your little one will experience in her first twelve months of life. As a parent you will find yourself saying and hearing things that used to sound cliché but now ring true: "Enjoy this time; they grow up so fast" or "They seem to grow up overnight." Indeed, your infant will have spurts in which she's literally growing overnight. One night you put your sweet little one down to sleep in a cozy one-piece pajama that fits just perfectly, and the next morning you wake up and the entire outfit seems to have shrunk.

Full-term infants tend to have growth spurts in predictable patterns. The first growth spurt happens shortly after a mother's milk volume increases and transitions from colostrum to mature milk—between three to seven days postpartum. After that, growth spurts fall into a pattern of the threes and sixes. You'll typically see growth spurts at three weeks, six weeks, three months, and six months. (For premature infants, this range can vary—some will fall into this predictable schedule, and some will have one all their own. Always use your infant's corrected age when determining appropriate behavior and milestones.)

While the end result of a growth spurt is exciting and fun to see, the growth spurt itself demands a great deal of resources from your infant and from you. Your infant will have a temporary increase in caloric needs, which will cause a shift in feeding and sleeping patterns. During a growth spurt, it's normal for an infant to suddenly begin to nurse fourteen to sixteen times a day with shorter breaks between nursing sessions. This means your baby will wake more often to feed. This is normal and won't last forever. Growth spurts typically last anywhere from three to five days, sometimes stretching to a week. I receive countless calls a week from mothers worried that their milk supply has suddenly dropped because their infant is "constantly nursing" and "never seems satisfied." Many mothers worry that during a growth spurt they simply won't have enough milk to meet their infant's high demands. Think back to the breastfeeding law of demand

and supply. Every time your infant nurses and "demands" milk, she is telling your body to make more milk. Put simply, your body will rise to the task and is ready to feed your infant at all times.

Growth spurts aren't physically demanding only on baby but on mom as well. Find a comfortable position like the side-lying position to nurse your infant. Growth spurts tend to happen in the early weeks and months when visitors are still plentiful. When friends and family stop by to see the baby, give them a task, whether it be unloading the dishwasher, grabbing you and your partner dinner from your favorite restaurant, or helping to fold an accumulating pile of clothes. Don't be afraid to ask for help and accept help as a parent, especially in these early months when much of your time and resources are dedicated to growing a healthy child. Lastly, in this moment, when you're tired and your infant seems to only want to nurse all day and all night, remember that this is temporary. In a couple of days it will pass and you'll see that hard work pay off in the form of chubbier cheeks and bigger smiles—it will seem that your baby has grown up overnight.

RETURNING TO WORK OR SCHOOL

Working outside the home can present a unique set of challenges to the modern breastfeeding mother. Before 1991, there was no consistently reliable means of milk expression for mothers beyond hand expression, and, therefore, infants had to be switched to formula out of necessity when the mother returned to work or other commitments. This isn't to say that hand expression isn't a valuable tool, but it's one that mothers need to practice and perfect in order to be effective, whereas pumping requires no practice. In this way, commercial breast pumps have completely changed the way we as a culture think about infant feeding during separations. While an electric breast pump is an indispensable tool to the working mother, it isn't perfect. Breast pumps can't mimic the suckling of an infant or draw milk from the breast as effectively as your infant can (for more on why you should always breastfeed rather than pump when it's possible, see page 75).

Pumping at work is protected under federal law. According to the Department of Labor, the amended section 7 of the Fair Labor Standards Act (FLSA) requires that employers provide adequate break time for their employees to either breastfeed or express milk for their infant for one year after the child's birth. (Employers with exemptions from the requirements of section 7 may still be obligated to provide breaks under state laws.) Employers are also required to provide a safe location that can be used by breastfeeding mothers to express milk. The location must be a place other than a bathroom, shielded from view, and free from contact with other employees and the public.

Employees who are included under FLSA's overtime pay requirements are also entitled to breaks for breastfeeding. For employers who have fifty or fewer employees, they aren't required to follow the FLSA break-time requirements if complying with the law would lead to an undue hardship. This exemption is determined by evaluating the difficulty or expense of compliance for a specific employer. This difficulty may be associated with financial resources or the nature or structure of the employer's business.

Also, employers aren't required under the FLSA to compensate breastfeeding mothers for breaks taken for the purpose of expressing milk. However, many women wear a hands-free bustier when pumping to allow them the ability to do a job-related task that doesn't require major movement, such as checking and replying to work emails—I've done my fair share of conference calls while pumping! If working while pumping isn't desirable or possible, then simply take this time to relax. In fact, finding something to do to distract yourself while pumping can help to increase milk output, since you're allowing you mind to relax and focus on something other than how much milk you'll produce. Set a timer for fifteen to twenty minutes, pull up a good book or your favorite series on Netflix, and enjoy this short break in the day for yourself.

From a personal standpoint, I can tell you there are very few places I haven't pumped. My journey into motherhood began while I was a student finishing my master's thesis, working outside the home, and working on my intern practicum hours for both my dietitian and IBCLC credentials. Needless to say, I was on the road a lot and found myself pumping just about any place I could find with an outlet. I've pumped everywhere from tattoo parlors and storage closets to churches and, more times than I can count,

my car. I've even pumped in the back of a classroom full of students with a little curtain separating me from the class so I could pump without missing class. The life of a breastfeeding mother can be hectic, but taking the time wherever you are to stop, relax, and pump is important not only for the nutritional needs of your child but also to allow you the freedom to breastfeed while working.

Because breast pumps typically yield a much smaller output of milk than nursing does, some mothers might have to pump twice to get one bottle's worth of milk for their little ones. This is normal. While normal, it does not solve the practical problem that many mothers simply don't have the time in a day to pump enough to fill three to four bottles. This is where galactagogues and lactogenic foods come in (see Chapter 9). They are an incredibly useful tool in helping to boost your breast milk without trying to find a way to squeeze six to eight pumping sessions into your day and night.

Finding a caregiver who is experienced and comfortable with paced bottle-feedings is important. Propping an infant's bottle without someone holding it for her is incredibly unsafe, as is leaving a child unattended with a bottle to feed.

During a bottle-feeding session, an infant should be held close to the body, and the bottle should not be placed into the baby's mouth until she opens her mouth up wide, just as she would when latching on at the breast. From this point, you can now slowly insert the bottle into the baby's mouth, continuing to encourage a wide mouth and strong latch. Allow baby to suckle for a bit (around thirty seconds to a minute) and then tilt the bottle nipple down so that no air is passing through the nipple but also no milk is flowing. Hold the bottle in this position for another ten to thirty seconds and then proceed to continue the feed. Continue in this pattern until the feeding is complete. Alternatively, you can stop the feeding after every ounce and distract her by burping or playing for a bit and then returning to feeding. An infant should never be put flat on her back to bottle-feed, and the bottle should always be parallel with the floor.

Another common pitfall is trying to provide more milk than is necessary because an infant is being overfed. Some mothers who have a strong oversupply might be able to consistently pump enough milk to overfeed a baby, but most will not. Overfeeding is synonymous with bottle-feeding. Bottle-feeding is a passive form of eating, while breastfeeding is a very active one that requires the full participation of the child. Because overfeeding is so common in bottle-fed babies, it's often seen as the norm in our culture. Infants are frequently seen with an eight-ounce bottle filled all the way to the top, when, in fact, an infant's maximum stomach capacity is only five ounces, and most breastfed babies only need three to four ounces in a bottle to meet their caloric and nutritional needs. While formula-fed babies tend to have feeding schedules and ranges that follow their weight or their age, breastfeeding babies do not. Unlike formula, breast milk changes with the baby, and your little one's ability to digest and absorb nutrients from your milk also changes. Because of this, your infant does not need to take in a larger quantity of breast milk as she gets older, because the qualities of the breast milk change. If your infant is consistently drinking more than four ounces of expressed breast milk in a bottle, then it's time to begin working on a plan to slow down the pace of feedings to allow time for your infant's stomach to tell her brain that it's full.

WELCOME BACK, AUNT FLO!

Lactation-induced amenorrhea is a phenomenon that occurs in the weeks, months, and sometimes years postpartum in which a woman does not ovulate or have a menstrual cycle while breastfeeding. For some women, their menstrual cycle returns within three months postpartum, and for others, eighteen months postpartum. Researchers are beginning to find clues as to why this varies so widely. Over time, serum prolactin levels begin to decline in a breastfeeding mother. Once this occurs, a mother's milk supply is highly dependent on her infant's ability to transfer milk effectively. Once prolactin levels begin to decline, if milk removal also declines then milk supply will decrease dramatically. However, research has shown that prolactin levels tend to remain high in mothers whose infants nurse frequently (on demand) throughout the day. If this frequent removal of milk occurs, then prolactin levels can stay high for eighteen months or more.[1]

Anytime nursing decreases to levels that the body recognizes as weaning (typically under eight nursing sessions a day), blood levels of prolactin begin to decrease and levels of luteinizing hormone and estradiol sharply increase, signaling to the body that it's time to start ovulating again.[2] Luteinizing hormone's specific job is to signal ovulation, and estradiol is the strongest of the three types of estrogen that women naturally produce. Once this hormonal cascade begins, ovulation typically returns in fourteen to thirty days, although it might take an additional cycle for a woman's period to return.

When a woman's menstrual cycle returns, this typically signals the beginning of hormone-mediated milk supply changes throughout the month. Most mothers report that one to two days before the onset of their period as well as the first two to three days of their period, their milk supply drops. In addition to a drop in supply, the hormones related to menstruation also cause changes in the milk's taste. Most infants will compensate for this change by nursing more often, while others unaccustomed to the taste of the milk will nurse less often. This drop in milk supply is normal and transient. Typically, a mother will still make enough milk to nourish her child effectively. However, for women who are separated from their infants during menstruation, perhaps after returning to school or working outside the home, it can be distressing to try to cope with lower pumping output for nearly a week at a time.

Shatavari is a lactogenic herb commonly used by women throughout India from puberty to menopause for reproductive health. Shatavari appears to exert its most powerful lactogenic effects during menstruation and has been noted to help many women maintain a normal milk supply throughout their periods[3] (for more on shatavari, see page 111). Many women also find that taking 500 to 1000 mg of a calcium/magnesium supplement at night three days before and throughout their period helps. While there's currently no clinical evidence that backs up this practice, there's a large body of anecdotal evidence that shows that calcium/magnesium supplementation might help with the supply slumps that coincide with the return of the menstrual cycle.

STRESS

Stress is a broad term covering a variety of physiological and psychological experiences that manifest themselves in different ways. Psychological stress can come from a hectic day at work, caring for an ailing loved one, or simply running late. Physiological or physical stress can come from an illness or strain that has been put on the body, causing it to function in a suboptimal way.

In many cultures there's a widely held belief that stress spoils a mother's breast milk. While we know that this isn't true, the origins of this folk belief are based in fact. When a mother is under a great deal of stress, her milk supply typically begins to decline. In some women this decline is rapid, and in some it is a slow process. Stress inhibits the release of oxytocin, which is an essential component in the milk eject reflex referred to as letdowns; because of this, an infant may take longer than usual to get the milk she needs.[4]

Ashwagandha is an herb traditionally used in ayurvedic medicine for the management of stress. Many breastfeeding mothers find it to be a beneficial herb to boost milk supply during stressful times. For more information on the use of ashwagandha in breastfeeding mothers, see page 117.

MALNUTRITION

I hate to admit it, but even I fell into the malnutrition trap while nursing my firstborn. As a dietitian and lactation consultant, I knew how important nutrition is to maintaining a healthy milk supply. But as a first-time mother balancing motherhood, building a new business, and writing, I found myself putting the needs of everyone above myself. I would make beautiful nutritious meals from scratch for my family, yet, somehow, I wasn't eating enough or as often as I should have been. After twelve months of experiencing an oversupply that allowed me to donate gallons and gallons of milk for low-birth-weight preemies, I found myself with barely enough milk to fill a bottle. When I spoke with one of my mentors (a breastfeeding support group leader for over thirty years and one of the first in the country to take the IBCLC exam), she told me unequivocally that I was wasting away. It was clear I wasn't nourishing myself, and my low milk supply was the evidence of that lack of self-care.

I share this story to remind you that we are all human, and as mothers many of us share the same struggles. Every day I find myself sitting across from mothers—new and seasoned, working and stay-at-home, young and mature—and over and over again I hear of mothers putting the needs of all others before their own. When it comes to nourishing our bodies, you help your child by helping yourself.

This isn't to say that trying to lose weight while breastfeeding is completely off the table. I talk at length about how to properly lose weight while maintaining a healthy milk supply on pages 93–95. However, any diet that is incredibly restrictive in calories is likely to be a detriment to your milk supply. While breastfeeding, your body is burning up to an additional 600 calories a day. This means that your caloric needs during lactation are nearly double that of what they were when you were pregnant. This also means that if you aren't nourishing yourself properly throughout the day, your body will quickly become calorie deficit. Not only can an unhealthy and unsafe level of weight loss occur, but it also becomes increasingly difficult to maintain a healthy milk supply.

If your milk supply has dropped and you suspect malnutrition is the culprit, then I highly recommend reading through the next part carefully to learn about the ins and outs of a healthy diet for the breastfeeding mother. Many lactogenic foods are also foods that are high in nutrients and, in the right balance, will help to meet the unique nutrient needs of a breastfeeding woman. In addition to improving the quality of your diet, supplementing with lactogenic herbs such as moringa and shatavari in addition to lactogenic foods like oatmeal and barley will be essential to helping your body recover from the stress of malnutrition.

PART THREE

Breastfeeding and Nutrition

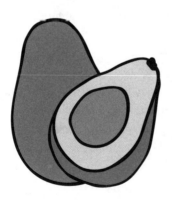

NOURISHING YOUR BODY

There's a commonly held belief that a mother's diet can positively or negatively influence the quality of her milk—that if she eats nothing but cheeseburgers and fries, her milk won't have adequate nutrients for her child, and if she eats a perfectly balanced meal filled with fresh organic vegetables, lean proteins, and whole grains, she'll make the highest-quality milk. As a dietitian, I would love to tell you that eating the perfect diet is the key to having the highest-quality milk, but that simply isn't true. However, eating a healthy, well-balanced diet will allow you to be the healthiest version of yourself and increase your quality of life.

During both pregnancy and lactation, your little one will take nutrients from you preferentially. This means that if your body has to make a choice between nourishing your heart with omega-3 fatty acids or using those same omega-3 fatty acids to help build your baby's central nervous system, your body will choose your baby. If your body has to choose between utilizing vitamin C to help heal a cut in your skin or to help strengthen your infant's skin—your body will choose your baby. Therefore, having a well-balanced and healthy diet isn't important only for the health of your little one, but for yours, as well. You want to ensure that your body has enough nutrients to go around so that both you and your baby can be well nourished and healthy.

Remember: Your body can't give your baby what it doesn't have. Vital nutrients are stored in nearly every cell of your body, so you have a large reserve to pull from to help your body create good-quality milk. This chapter is your crash course in nutrition for the breastfeeding mother.

MANAGING FOOD ALLERGIES AND BREASTFEEDING

Parents often come to my office worried that their family history of food allergies will be passed on to their children and wonder what they can do to prevent this. Your first line of defense to reduce the risk of food allergies in your little ones is to breastfeed them! Breastfeeding has been shown to significantly reduce the risk of food allergies as well as other allergic manifestations like eczema and respiratory allergies.[1] Additionally, current evidence doesn't support a mother restricting her diet of potentially allergenic foods during lactation (or pregnancy) as a preventive measure against food allergies.[2]

If you experience food allergies or sensitivities yourself and are worried about leaving these foods out of your diet while you breastfeed, you should know that nearly any type of eating preference or preexisting food allergy can be accommodated into the diet of a breastfeeding mother. As long as the four main components of a healthy, well-balanced meal are present within your diet, you're likely on the right track. These four components are lean proteins (including beans, nuts, and seeds), vegetables, fruits, and whole grains. In general, you should fill half your plate with vegetables or fruit (preferably more vegetables than fruit), one fourth of your plate with protein, and one fourth of your plate with whole grains or starchy vegetables.

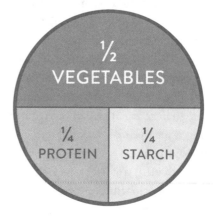

MATERNAL ENERGY NEEDS DURING PREGNANCY AND LACTATION

Many mothers believe that pregnancy is a time when they can eat whatever they want without consequence. However, this is a false and sometimes dangerous myth that leads many new and expectant mothers into my office due to pre- and postnatal complications associated with excess weight gain during pregnancy. Excess weight gain during pregnancy increases the risk of maternal mortality, gestational diabetes, thromboembolism, preeclampsia, and postpartum hemorrhage.[3] Excess weight gain during pregnancy also increases the risk of cesarean delivery, complications during cesarean delivery, and longer hospital stays.[4] The risk associated with excessive antepartum weight gain does not stop with the mother. Infants born to women with excess weight gain during pregnancy are at risk of being born large for their gestational age, developing reactive hypoglycemia, and having an increased risk of fetal abnormalities as well as stillbirth and miscarriage.[5] Conversely, while it is important to not gain excessive weight while pregnant, it is also important to not gain too little weight. Inadequate weight gain in the second and third trimesters of pregnancy nearly doubles the risk of preterm birth.[6]

Calorie needs during pregnancy are relatively low when compared to those of a breastfeeding mother. During the first trimester of pregnancy, a woman's energy needs remain constant, meaning no additional calories are needed. In the second and third trimesters, energy needs increase to approximately 300 additional calories a day, which is equivalent to half a peanut butter and jelly sandwich and a small piece of fruit.

Consider these general guidelines for pregnancy weight gain:

PREPREGNANCY WEIGHT	RECOMMENDED WEIGHT GAIN[7]
Underweight (BMI less than 18.5)	28 to 40 pounds (about 13 to 18 kilograms)
Normal weight (BMI 18.5 to 24.9)	25 to 35 pounds (about 11 to 16 kilograms)
Overweight (BMI 25 to 29.9)	15 to 25 pounds (about 7 to 11 kilograms)
Obese (BMI 30 or 39.9)	11 to 20 pounds (about 5 to 9 kilograms)
Morbidly obese (BMI 40 or more)	0 to 10 pounds (about 0 to 4 kilograms)

Women who stick within the recommended weight gain ranges for pregnancy tend to have the healthiest birth outcomes and lose weight faster postpartum.[8] The reason mothers lose weight faster when they stick to the Institute of Medicine's recommended guidelines for weight gain is because they are only gaining what their infant needs to thrive and not excess fat stores. Here is a breakdown of what those extra 300 calories a day help build:

Baby:
7 to 8 pounds (about 3 to 3.5 kg)

Larger breasts:
2 pounds (about 1 kg)

Larger uterus:
2 pounds (about 1 kg)

Placenta:
1½ pounds (about 0.5 kg)

Amniotic fluid:
2 pounds (about 1 kg)

Increased blood volume:
3 to 4 pounds (about 1.5 to 2 kg)

Increased fluid volume:
3 to 4 pounds (about 1.5 to 2 kg)

Fat stores:
6 to 8 pounds (3 to 3.5 kg)

That's a total of 27 to 35 pounds (about 12 to 15.5 kg)!

The calorie needs of a breastfeeding mother are markedly higher than that of the average nonlactating female—breastfeeding is one of the rare times in a woman's life where she can eat an extra 500 to 600 calories a day and typically not gain weight! This is because on average a breastfeeding mother can burn up to 600 calories by breastfeeding alone. Breast milk contains 20 calories per ounce, which means for every ounce of breast milk you make, your body uses 20 calories. Since a breastfed baby will consume anywhere from 19 to 30 ounces of breast milk a day, breastfeeding mothers will burn 380 to 600 calories a day by breastfeeding. That's the equivalent of running at a moderate pace for about an hour! This is one of the reasons why breastfeeding mothers, overall, lose weight faster and go back to their prepregnancy weights at a faster rate than their nonbreastfeeding counterparts.[9]

LOSING WEIGHT WHILE BREASTFEEDING

We live in a culture that presses moms to "eat for two" while pregnant, which encourages poor eating habits during pregnancy, and then expects mothers to quickly return to their prepregnancy weight within weeks or months following the birth of their child. If a woman gains a healthy amount of weight during pregnancy, she will likely return to her prepregnancy weight within the first six months postpartum. However, this isn't an absolute for all women.

No matter what your BMI was prepregnancy or how much weight you gained while you were pregnant, weight loss should be pushed to the side for the first eight weeks after your child's birth. There are enough things to worry about and major adjustments to make in your journey into motherhood—try not to let weight be a source of stress. In the weeks and months after your baby is born, your body is going through the very first stages of healing and returning to its prepregnancy shape. Your uterus, which took forty weeks to grow, is decreasing back down to its original size in just about six weeks. Your breasts are going through myriad changes as they adjust to your infant's needs. Your muscles and bones are shifting back into place. Give yourself the time you need to heal!

Once you your body begins to feel restored, you can begin to think about trying to reach and maintain a healthy weight. Losing weight while breastfeeding is safe, as long as it's done with care. Rapid weight loss via extreme calorie restriction isn't safe for anyone, breastfeeding or not—severely limiting your calorie intake means you're severely limiting the nutrients you're consuming, as well. You also shouldn't take medicine for weight loss or go on a restrictive diet that severely limits or eliminates entire groups of foods, such as a liquid diet, low- or no-carb diet, no-fat diet, or diet that removes important foods like beans, nuts, or seeds. Losing weight by these methods or any method of rapid weight loss can cause a reduction in milk supply and put you at risk for nutrient deficiency. While on your weight-loss journey, remember that temporary changes will get you temporary results. You must make changes that can last a lifetime—and, let's be honest, no one is going a lifetime without carbs!

It's also important to note that fasting is never recommended for breastfeeding mothers, due to the potential for rapid weight loss and immediate cessation of the nutrient supply to the mother. Nearly all religious observances that have a fasting component exempt nursing mothers. Fasting in any form—via a liquid diet, total cessation of eating for a full twenty-four hours, or even fasting for part of the day—isn't recommended while breastfeeding and typically has a negative effect on milk supply.

Losing approximately 1 to 2 pounds (0.5 to 1 kg) a week is considered to be a safe rate of weight loss while breastfeeding.[10] It won't surprise you that weight loss through both diet modification and exercise is preferable to weight loss by diet modification alone, as weight loss by dieting alone tends to reduce a mother's lean muscle mass.[11] Exercise has been shown to have no negative effect on lactation and in some cases has been reported to improve lactation due to an increase in prolactin concentration during exercise.[12]

Studies have also demonstrated that mothers who nurse on demand for over six months have increased weight loss as well.[13] So continuing to nurse your child not only is beneficial to your child but can help you lose those last extra pounds!

MACRONUTRIENT NEEDS OF THE BREASTFEEDING WOMAN

Macronutrients are nutrients that are required in large quantities to sustain life. Carbohydrates, fats, and proteins are all macronutrients. Each has an important role in the health of the breastfeeding mother. The following are general guidelines for macronutrient needs while breastfeeding.

Carbohydrates

No one nutrient is more important than the next. Each plays a vital role in your health and milk production as well as in the health of your infant. Carbohydrates provide the most readily available form of energy to your body and are the main fuel source that your brain utilizes. Each organ system has a nutrient that it prefers as its main fuel source. For the brain, this is carbohydrates, specifically glucose. If you have ever felt a headache or started to feel unhappy or uneasy after skipping a meal, this is your brain telling you that it needs more glucose to function. This is also why if you skip a meal or allow yourself to get too hungry, your brain tells you to eat something with a readily available source of glucose—which for many people means grabbing the first cookie, cupcake, candy bar, or high-sugar food they can find. To prevent your body from getting to this point, keep healthy snacks with you and munch on them between meals. Healthy snacks include fruits, raw vegetables, whole grains, or lean proteins like nuts and seeds. In general, the recommended intake of carbohydrates for breastfeeding mothers is 210 grams a day, the highest need of any period in a woman's life. Of course there's some variation from person to person on exactly how many grams of carbohydrates you should consume in a day. Therefore, if you're concerned about your macronutrient intake while breastfeeding, I highly recommend that you consult a registered dietitian who specializes in maternal health to find out your specific needs.

Good Fats

As we previously discussed, every organ system has a nutrient that it prefers as its main fuel source. For the heart, that nutrient is fat. Without fat, the heart can't properly function. However, not all fats are beneficial to the heart. Saturated and trans fats promote cardiovascular disease, while omega-3 and omega-6 fatty acids and mono- and polyunsaturated fats promote cardiovascular health.

Unlike most nutrients, the type of fats that you eat directly affects the type of fats that are in your breast milk. If your diet is high in healthy fats such as those in plant-based oils, then your milk will have a high level of healthy fats in it. If your diet is high in unhealthy fats, such as those found in animals, your breast milk will have lower amounts of healthy fats. However, in both cases, your milk will still have fat, your infant will still grow and be healthy, and all the scientific evidence we have available shows us that, for the long and short term, breast milk is still the healthiest option for infants.

OMEGA-3 ESSENTIAL FATTY ACIDS

It's hard to escape the powerful allure of omega-3 fatty acids these days. They're being studied for just about every imaginable medical condition, and research has shown that they could be beneficial for such diseases and conditions as cancer, inflammatory bowel disease, lupus, rheumatoid arthritis, heart disease, stroke, postpartum depression, autism, and ADHD. Omega-3 fatty acids help control blood clotting and build cell membranes in the brain; therefore, the fatty acid content of your breast milk is vital to the development of the infant brain.[14]

Research shows that simply consuming omega-3 fatty acids through food or supplements isn't enough to positively influence fetal brain development. Rather, the ratio between omega-6 and omega-3 fatty acids in your diet is as paramount to brain development as the consumption of omega-3s alone (see the section on hemp seeds on page 117 for more on the 3:1 ratio). It's important to note this subtle change between the roles of omega-6s and omega-3s in pregnancy versus lactation. While the omega-6 to omega-3 ratio is important during pregnancy, studies have not yet demonstrated that a high omega-6 to omega-3 ratio has a negative impact on infant brain development postpartum.[15]

The adequate intake of omega-3 fatty acids has been set at 1.3 grams by the Institute of Medicine, with an acceptable macronutrient distribution range (AMDR) of 0.6 to 1.2 grams a day for breastfeeding women.

OMEGA-6 ESSENTIAL FATTY ACIDS

In general, Americans consume more omega-6 fatty acids than omega-3 fatty acids. The imbalance in consumption of these two fatty acids is central to research into the effects of overconsumption of omega-6 fatty acids on neurologic and cardiovascular health as well as the development of chronic disease. While consuming more omega-6 fatty acids than omega-3 fatty acids may be detrimental to one's health, this doesn't mean that omega-6 fatty acids are "bad." Omega-6 fatty acids are essential fatty acids, meaning that our bodies can't make them but they are essential to human health. Omega-6 fatty acids play an important role in brain function as well as normal growth and development. Omega-6 fatty acids help stimulate skin and hair growth, maintain bone health, regulate metabolism, and maintain reproductive health.

The adequate intake of omega-6 fatty acids has been set at 13 grams a day by the Institute of Medicine. To date there's no general recommended daily intake of omega-6 fatty acids.

Many foods contain both omega-3 and omega-6 essential fatty acids.

Below is a short list of some of the richest sources of each nutrient:

SOURCES OF OMEGA-3 FATTY ACIDS	SOURCES OF OMEGA-6 FATTY ACIDS
Flaxseed	Corn oil
Chia seed	Sunflower oil
Hemp seed	Peanut oil
Salmon	Poultry (specifically poultry fat)
Blue-green algae	Nuts/seeds
Walnuts	Mayonnaise
Canola oil	Salad dressing
Soybean oil	Vegetable oil

MONOUNSATURATED FATTY ACIDS AND POLYUNSATURATED FATTY ACIDS

Monounsaturated fatty acids (MUFAs) and polyunsaturated fatty acids (PUFAs) are also two very popular fats that we often hear about in the news in relation to heart health. Monounsaturated and polyunsaturated fats are fats that are typically liquid at room temperature but begin to turn solid when chilled. Olive oil is high in monounsaturated fats. You can do your own quick science experiment at home by putting a bottle of olive oil in the refrigerator. You'll notice that within minutes the oil becomes cloudy and starts to solidify. Both omega-3s and omega-6s are types of polyunsaturated fats.

SOURCES OF MONO-UNSATURATED FATTY ACIDS	SOURCES OF POLY-UNSATURATED FATTY ACIDS
Olive oil	Soybeans and soybean oil
Canola oil	Corn oil
Peanut oil	Sunflower seeds and sunflower oil
Safflower oil	Fatty fish (salmon, mackerel, herring, and trout)
Sesame oil	Walnuts
Avocado	Hemp

There's a significant positive effect from the consumption of PUFAs and MUFAs on the fat status of breast milk.[16] Intake of these healthy essential fatty acids affects the fatty acid profile of breast milk and, in turn, affects an infant's consumption of these vital fatty acids.

Protein

Western culture puts a great deal of emphasis on protein consumption. However, the majority of Americans eat two to three times the amount of protein they need, and this can lead to a variety of ailments, including dehydration, headaches, calcium loss, abnormal heart rhythms, low blood sugar and pressure, swollen limbs, liver damage, and stomach issues, as well increasing your risk of diabetes and osteoporosis.[17]

The protein needs of a pregnant woman and breastfeeding mother are nearly identical. Both women need on average approximately 25 additional grams of protein a day. On average this is approximately 71 grams of protein a day for a mother with a healthy prepregnancy BMI. However, there's significant variation based on height and prepregnancy weight. It's best to consult with a registered dietitian well versed in maternal nutrition to calculate what your protein needs are while breastfeeding.

MICRONUTRIENT NEEDS OF THE BREASTFEEDING WOMAN

Micronutrients are nutrients that are required in small quantities to sustain life. Micronutrients are commonly referred to as vitamins and minerals, but we're learning that micronutrients are not just major vitamins and minerals but also biologically active components of plants called phytonutrients and phytochemicals, as well as plant hormones like phytoestrogens. It's no surprise that the majority of foods that have high levels of the micronutrients that breastfeeding mothers need the most are also foods that have been used as galactagogues for generations in cultures around the world. While we are just starting to uncover the science of lactogenic foods and how they work, sages, medicine women, village elders, midwives, and even lactation consultants have been using these foods for centuries to help mothers improve the quality and quantity of breast milk. Before I go into some of these lactogenic foods in the next chapter, here's what you need to know about the vitamins and minerals important to breastfeeding.

Vitamins and Minerals

For breastfeeding women, only a small handful of vitamins and minerals have recommended daily intakes (RDAs) substantially greater than the average nonbreastfeeding woman. Only vitamin A, vitamin C, chromium, copper, and iodine are needed in quantities nearly double that of a nonlactating woman. However, obtaining more of these vitamins and minerals can be easily done through diet alone.

VITAMIN A

Vitamin A plays a major role in eye development and vision, supports cell growth and immune function, and is key in the formation of the heart, lungs, and kidneys. Green leafy vegetables, as well as plants that have red- or orange-hued flesh, are high in vitamin A and are regarded as galactagogues in many cultures. Sweet potatoes, carrots, kale, butternut squash, romaine lettuce, dried apricots, cantaloupe, and mango are among the richest sources of vitamin A. Breastfeeding mothers need 1,300 mcg (4,333 IU) of vitamin A a day, which is the equivalent of a third of a small baked sweet potato. See pages 115–116 for more on the possible lactogenic properties of leafy greens and reddish vegetables.

VITAMIN C

Vitamin C is vital for your baby's growing bones and tissue and will help you fight disease. Excellent food sources of vitamin C include broccoli, bell peppers, brussels sprouts, strawberries, mustard greens, kiwifruit, papaya, kale, cabbage, romaine lettuce, turnip greens, oranges, cantaloupe, summer squash, grapefruit, pineapple, chard, tomatoes, and collard greens. Nursing moms should get 120 mg of vitamin C a day, which is equivalent to one kiwi or a half cup of strawberries and a half cup of pineapple.

CHROMIUM

Our bodies don't need a lot of chromium each day (only 25 mcg for nonlactating women and 45 mcg for lactating ones), but it has many important jobs, including helping to control the metabolism of carbohydrates, proteins, and fats. Brewer's yeast, broccoli, mushrooms, oatmeal, prunes, nuts, asparagus, whole grains, cereals, and red wine are all rich sources of chromium. Not coincidentally, brewer's yeast, mushrooms, oatmeal, nuts, and whole grains are all popular lactogenic foods used throughout the world for their milk-making properties.

COPPER

Copper is a trace mineral, meaning it is only needed in very small amounts. Eating just 1.3 mg a day is all a breastfeeding mother needs to meet her daily nutrient needs for copper. Seafood such as spirulina (a seaweed often found in powder form) and oysters, as well as whole grains, kale, shiitake mushrooms, sesame seeds, sunflower seeds, nuts, beans, fermented soy products (tempeh and miso), and dried fruit are all good sources of copper.

IODINE

Iodine is the principle building block of two important thyroid hormones—triiodothyronine and thyroxine, commonly referred to as T3 and T4. These hormones help maintain thyroid function, which affects your body's metabolic processes, protein synthesis, and enzyme activity, just to name a few. Seaweed is the most abundant natural source of iodine. Iodized salt is the next best source of iodine in the diet. If you use sea salt or kosher salt, look out for ones fortified with iodine to ensure that you are getting enough of this important nutrient. To read more about your thyroid's relationship to breastfeeding, see page 44.

Other Micronutrient Concerns

VITAMIN D

Vitamin D is also known as the "sunshine" vitamin because our bodies synthesize it directly from unobstructed exposure to the sun. Vitamin D is not naturally found in any appreciable amounts from food sources. For many years the scientific community thought that breast milk was naturally low in vitamin D, but new studies have shown that maternal vitamin D exposure directly affects the vitamin D in her milk. In other words, like fats, the amount of vitamin D in your milk will vary based on your intake or exposure. Women who supplemented with 6,400 IU of vitamin D a day had the highest level of vitamin D in their milk and were able to meet their infant's recommended vitamin D needs with breast milk alone.

EAT LESS IRON

If you were loading up on iron during your pregnancy, good news:

Breastfeeding women have drastically lower iron needs than that of a pregnant woman, so you can ditch those prenatal vitamins. In pregnancy a woman needs 27 mg of iron a day, while during lactation she only requires 9 mg of iron a day. In fact, nursing mothers have even lower iron needs than nonbreastfeeding women aged eighteen to fifty.

WORRY LESS ABOUT CALCIUM

Many people believe that calcium needs are higher during pregnancy and lactation. This is a pretty logical conclusion—it seems like it would take a lot of extra calcium to grow an entire human being—however, the calcium needs of a pregnant or lactating woman are the same as a nonpregnant or nonlactating woman, at just 1,000 mg a day.

Specific Micronutrient Needs

Wondering how much of each specific nutrient you're supposed to be getting? On the next page is a complete table of the micronutrient needs of a breastfeeding woman.

NUTRIENT	RECOMMENDED DIETARY ALLOWANCE (RDA)
Vitamin A	1,300 mcg or 4,333 IU
Vitamin C	120 mg
Vitamin D	15 mcg or 600 IU
Vitamin E	19 mg
Vitamin K	90 mcg
Thiamin	1.4 mg
Riboflavin	1.6 mg
Niacin	17 mg
Vitamin B6	2 mg
Folate	500 mcg
Vitamin B12	2.8 mcg
Pantothenic Acid	7 mg
Biotin	35 mcg
Choline	550 mg
Calcium	1,000 mg

NUTRIENT	RECOMMENDED DIETARY ALLOWANCE (RDA)
Chromium	45 mcg
Copper	1.3 mg
Fluoride	3 mg
Iodine	290 mcg
Iron	9 mg
Magnesium	320 mg
Manganese	2.6 mg
Molybdenum	50 mcg
Phosphorus	700 mg
Selenium	70 mcg
Zinc	12 mg
Potassium	5,100 mg
Sodium	1,500 mg
Chloride	2,300 mg

BOOSTING YOUR BREAST MILK THROUGH FOODS AND HERBS

When it comes to low milk supply, most moms want to know one thing—what is going to be the magic pill that makes their milk supply come back or the right herb, root, or plant that ensures they will maintain a healthy milk supply. But a low milk supply can be caused by a wide variety of things, and, while nutrient-rich and lactogenic foods and herbs work well in boosting your breast milk supply, they'll only be a Band-Aid covering up the larger problem underneath that has caused low milk supply in the first place. Make sure to read through Part II to see whether there's an easy, non-nutrition-related solution to your low milk supply, and consult an International Board Certified Lactation Consultant, who can be incredibly useful in helping to determine your specific causes for low milk supply if they aren't immediately evident.

So many women walk into my office with bags full of herbs and supplements, desperate to increase their milk supply. As tempting as it might be to open up your online shopping cart and start filling it up with a bottle of every herb listed in this section, I would advise against it. In the next chapter, I talk a bit more specifically about which herbs to use depending on the origin of your milk supply issue, but, for now, there are two important things to remember—treat supplemental herbs like medication, and go slow. Because herbs are natural, many people assume that they carry no side effects; however, most do. In this chapter, I will discuss some of the side effects associated with each herb and lactogenic food, if any, as well as explain how each lactogenic food and herb helps boost your milk supply.

Along with foods shown in studies to have lactogenic effects, I'll discuss some that are traditionally considered lactogenic but have not been proven as such, as well as superfoods that will help nourish a breastfeeding mother. The chapter ends with a list of foods to avoid for their antilactogenic properties.

LACTOGENIC FOODS

Galactagogue, lactagogue, and lactogenic all refer to a broad class of medicines and foods (specifically edible plants and herbs) that increase the production of milk. Lactogenic foods and herbs are used to help promote a healthy and robust milk supply in not only humans but livestock as well. Nearly every culture in the world has its own beloved galactagogue used for generations to help nourish breastfeeding mothers. In India, women have used fenugreek seed and shatavari as galactagogues for centuries, while Mayan women used an herb called *ixbut*, native to Guatemala, to induce and promote lactation.

Edible plants and herbs are complex entities made up of phytonutrients, phytochemicals, and macro- and micronutrients. Science is just beginning to understand the role that phytonutrients and phytochemicals play in our overall health as well as in milk production. Phytochemicals and phytonutrients are broad terms referring to biologically active components of plants. Some commonly known phytochemicals are polyphenols, resveratrol, and carotenoids. To date, thousands of phytochemicals have been discovered by researchers; however, we still don't have a full understanding of what even a small handful of these phytochemicals do and why they benefit our health. For this reason, the mechanisms behind most lactogenic foods and herbs are still unknown.

We can, however, look at the compounds that we do know of in these foods and try to gain a better understanding of why they increase milk production and promote not only a healthy quantity but also quality of milk. Research has been conducted on many foods and herbs traditionally thought of as lactogenic, and scientific and clinical proof of their milk-making properties has been found. I've included here the most well-established lactogenic foods and herbs and the recommended daily amounts that have been shown to have a positive effect on milk supply. For delicious recipes that use these amazing foods, check out the Recipes section. For more on which lactogenic foods and herbs you should begin with, see page 130.

Barley and Malt

For more than a century, American, European, African, and Middle Eastern cultures have regarded beer as a galactagogue. However, research has shown that alcohol inhibits milk production and thus decreases milk supply (more about this on page 119). As with most old wives' tales and traditional cultural remedies, the basis for the use of beer as a galactagogue does have some science behind it. Research has shown that a component of beer, barley, is actually what is responsible for its perceived lactogenic properties.[1] Barley is the richest dietary source of beta-glucan, a polysaccharide that has been shown to increase prolactin levels in both humans and animals.[2] Readily available in the United States, barley is often used in soups and stews.

Malting is a process by which grains are germinated to release malting enzymes that convert the grain into sugar. In the case of barley malt, the enzyme diastase converts barley into a sweet, syrupy malt. Barley malt contains the same lactogenic polysaccharide, beta-glucan, as barley. In animal studies, barley malt and malt extracts have been shown to trigger the release of prolactin and increase circulating prolactin levels.[3]

You can purchase barley malt syrup online or at a health or specialty store. However, make sure to read the label of your malt carefully, as high-fructose or regular corn syrup is often used to dilute and sweeten commercially available barley malt syrup. Only buy malt that's made from 100 percent barley with no added fillers or sweeteners. Not sure how to use malt? Try Chocolate Malt Milk (page 140) or Peanut Butter Malted Cookies (page 215).

Oats

Oats are the most commonly used lactogenic food in the United States, and case studies and anecdotal evidence suggest that oats do have the robust lactogenic properties we have attributed to them. While the exact reason for oats' lactogenic power is unknown, researchers have been able to isolate various components of the grain that are believed to contribute to increased prolactin levels and milk supply. After barley, oats have a higher concentration of dietary beta-glucan than any other food.[4]

Other Whole Grains

Whole grains such as barley, oats, whole wheat, and brown rice are all rich in beta-glucan, that extraordinary prolactin-boosting polysaccharide. Whole wheat flour is such an integral part of the American diet that it's difficult to pinpoint whole wheat alone as a lactogenic food. The same is true of rice, specifically brown rice. Rice is a staple food not only in the Americas but around the world. In some cultures, rice is prepared with at least two daily meals. For this reason, whole wheat flour and rice have been overlooked in the research on galactagogues. When choosing a type of wheat flour or rice to purchase, remember that only 100 percent whole-grain wheat and brown rice are good sources of beta-glucan. White flour and white rice contain little to no beta-glucan.

Moringa

Moringa is known by many names all around the world. Its scientific name is *Moringa oleifera*, but it's commonly known as the horseradish tree (named for the bark's horseradish flavor), ben oil tree (the name of the oil made from its pods), drumstick tree, tree of life, miracle tree, and *mulanggay*, just to name a few. Moringa is cultivated in numerous countries, including the Philippines, India, Madagascar, Namibia, Angola, Kenya, Ethiopia, Pakistan, Bangladesh, Afghanistan, and Somalia. Throughout the Philippines and India, moringa is fed to nursing mothers in the form of a soup to ensure a healthy milk supply. Moringa leaf powder has been used to treat cases of anemia in pregnant and breastfeeding women in underdeveloped countries, either alone or in addition to ferrous sulfate supplements (depending on the severity of the anemia).[5] It is also used worldwide to help prevent and treat malnutrition (for more on the risks of becoming malnourished as a breastfeeding mother, see pages 85–87).

Moringa's seeds are very inexpensive and easy to harvest, the plant is drought-resistant, it grows quickly, and every part of the tree can be eaten. The leaves are the most widely studied part of the tree; they contain more than four times the amount of vitamin A found in carrots and nearly seven times the vitamin C of oranges.[6] They are also rich sources of B vitamins, calcium, iron, magnesium, phosphorus, zinc, copper, and potassium.[7]

While use of the pods of the moringa tree for breastfeeding mothers hasn't been studied, they are also traditionally used as a lactogenic food. The pods of the moringa tree have a complete amino acid profile, making these a rich source of protein.[8] The pods are particularly high in two amino acids, arginine and histidine, that are especially beneficial for infant growth. The pods are traditionally eaten like green peas or fried.

Moringa's lactogenic effects appear to come from its impact on the anterior pituitary gland. Clinical studies have shown that moringa significantly increases prolactin levels in women taking 250 mg capsules of dried moringa leaves once or twice a day.[9] This increase in prolactin levels was seen as early as forty-eight hours after starting to take them, and the effects were maintained for four months in clinical studies.[10] While some women reported an increase in their milk production in as little as twenty-four hours after initiating 250 mg of moringa daily, clinical data shows that there's a significant increase in breast milk volume by day seven.[11] When mothers who were exclusively pumping for preterm infants began using moringa, a significant increase in breast-milk volume was seen in four to five days.[12] The use of moringa has also been shown to significantly increase the weight and height of infants whose mothers were ingesting the leaves in whole or capsule form.[13] The typical dosage of moringa ranges from 250 mg a day to up to 700 mg a day.[14]

Unlike many other lactogenic herbs, moringa appears to have a clean safety profile on par with eating any other type of green leafy vegetable, making it one of the safest lactogenic herbs available today.[15] It's commonly available in the United States in powder form and can be found online and at health food stores.

Brewer's Yeast

Brewer's yeast is a by-product of the beer-making process and is often used as a nutritional supplement due to its high content of B vitamins, iron, protein, chromium, and selenium. While other components of beer such as barley and barley malt have been researched as galactagogues in humans, brewer's yeast has not. There are some animal studies that show that when a lactating animal's diet is fortified with brewer's yeast, the offspring of these mammals gain weight more efficiently and are healthier overall.[16] Studies have attributed this phenomenon to the improved nutritional status of the mother.[17]

Brewer's yeast is very bitter, so look for a brand that has "reduced bitterness." Brewer's yeast does pass readily into breast milk, and anecdotal evidence shows that, in some babies, this can cause gas and fussiness. When adding brewer's yeast to recipes, you typically have to compensate by adding a great deal of sugar to mask its bitter flavor. As a dietitian, I am always looking to reduce the intake of added sugars rather than increasing them, so I typically do not recommend much, if any, brewer's yeast for lactation support.

There is no clinically established dosage of brewer's yeast for lactation support. Generally, 500 to 1,000 mg a day of brewer's yeast in tablet form is thought to be the most effective. However, as I previously noted, there is an increased risk of gassiness in infants when mothers ingest brewer's yeast, and this risk is greater when it is taken in supplement form and not derived from food.

Fenugreek

As the use of lactogenic foods and herbs in the United States increases, so does the word-of-mouth reputation of certain herbs. One herb has emerged as the rock star of lactogenic herbs in the United States, and that is fenugreek. It has been used in India and some parts of the Middle East for generations as a powerful galactagogue. In fact, it's one of the oldest medicinal plants in recorded history.[18] While it is an incredibly popular herb, it is often used incorrectly, at the wrong dose, and with disregard for its side effects.

In my clinical practice, many mothers have a great deal of success increasing their milk supply with fenugreek supplements in combination with improved methods of nursing or milk expression (see Chapter 6). Fenugreek exerts its effect as a galactagogue by increasing prolactin levels.[19] Clinical studies have tried to identify the exact dosage that exerts therapeutic effects as well as the mechanism by which this herb works to increase milk production, but the evidence is still inconclusive.[20] Anecdotal accounts and case studies using fenugreek at a dosage of 1.16 g to 1.22 g three times a day have shown improvement in milk production and increased prolactin levels.[21] Fenugreek is also used in Chinese, Indian, and North African forms of natural medicine as an adjunct treatment for type 1 and type 2 diabetes, cardiovascular disease, and a variety of other chronic illnesses. Studies have shown that fenugreek can aid in lowering blood glucose levels as well as cholesterol.[22] Because of this, individuals who are currently under a physician's care for type 1 or 2 diabetes or hypocholesterolemia should consult with a physician before starting fenugreek to ensure there are no cross-reactions with current medications or therapies.

The most common side effect of fenugreek use is diarrhea and a (harmless) maple syrup smell to sweat and urine. There's also a possible cross-allergy reaction for those who are allergic to plants in the Asteraceae/Compositae family as well as peanuts, chickpeas, soybeans, and green peas.[23]

Milk Thistle

In addition to its use as a galactagogue, milk thistle is used as a natural and adjunct treatment for liver diseases as well as for cancer prevention. It's believed that compounds called flavonolignans in this appropriately named herb are the active ingredients that promote milk production in breastfeeding mothers.[24] Although milk thistle has been used for health for more than two thousand years, we are just beginning to get a full understanding of the role that flavonolignans play in health. Current evidence shows that in pill form, 420 mg a day is the most likely therapeutic dose of this herb. To achieve this same dosage via a homemade tea, the herb must be consumed at least two to three times a day.[25] If you have allergies to ragweed or any plant in the ragweed family, use of milk thistle isn't recommended due to a cross-reaction with the allergen. Additionally, there's the possibility that this herb increases the circulating levels of some statin (cholesterol-lowering) drugs, and it might also decrease blood levels of estrogen.[26]

Blessed thistle and milk thistle are often used interchangeably as lactogenic herbs, and sometimes it's even mistakenly said that blessed thistle is more effective than milk thistle. However, blessed thistle has no clinical evidence to support its use and very little anecdotal evidence that it can be used as a stand-alone herb for increased milk volume.

Shatavari

Shatavari (*Asparagus racemosus*) is a lactogenic herb commonly used throughout India from puberty to menopause for reproductive health. It's most often found in the United States in pill form in health food stores or online. The actual *Asparagus racemosus* plant is typically found in India, Australia, and parts of Africa, where it has been used for generations as a galactagogue and an herbal tonic for a variety of women's health issues

such as fertility and menstrual cycle regulation. Shatavari is used extensively in ayurvedic medicine as an antidysenteric, diuretic, aphrodisiac, and antispasmodic herb.

Chemical analysis of the root of *Asparagus racemosus* has found that it contains both cholesterol-reducing compounds and powerful antioxidants, and it has properties that make it effective against protozoa and other microbes, tumors, and some premature contractions.[27] Both animal and human studies have shown an increase in prolactin levels and milk yield with the administration of oral shatavari with a therapeutic dose of 60 mg per kg of body weight per day, in the form of capsules given three times during the day.[28] Shatavari appears to exert its most powerful lactogenic effects during menstruation and has been noted to help many women maintain a normal milk supply throughout their periods.[29] (See page 84 for more about menstruating while breastfeeding.)

Torbangun

The leaves of the torbangun plant (*Coleus amboinicus* [Lour.]) have been used throughout Indonesia for hundreds of years as a galactagogue. Small studies have shown that torbangun in supplemental form does increase milk supply; however, it doesn't reach maximum effect until two to three weeks, unlike other herbal galactagogues that only take a week or less.[30] In Indonesia, women typically consume the herb for at least four weeks.[31] Torbangun is difficult to find in the United States but may be available at some specialty markets and online retailers.

Goat's Rue

Goat's rue (*Galega officinalis*) is a popular lactogenic herb used throughout Europe. However, there's a lack of clinical evidence about the use of this herb as a stand-alone galactagogue. Most studies that show an increase in circulating prolactin levels with goat's rue were done in conjunction with another herb such as milk thistle or fenugreek.[32] It appears that when goat's rue is combined with other high-antioxidant lactogenic herbs such as fennel seed (see next page) it exerts its highest lactogenic effect;[33] to date, there haven't been any studies showing that the small amount of

goat's rue that would be used in food preparation would be enough to increase milk supply. Because of this, there isn't a standard, clinically studied dosage for goat's rue, but in clinical practice a once-daily dose of a 300 to 350 mg goat's rue supplement is considered safe and well tolerated by most women. Goat's rue is a flowering herb and not readily available in the United States in whole plant form, but it can be found in supplement form in specialty stores and online.

Papaya

In Asian cultures, papaya has long been used as a galactagogue. Both the ripe fruit and the unripened green papaya have reported lactogenic properties, whether you're eating them raw or making them into dishes like papaya salad or Thai sour soup. While papaya has been used for centuries as a galactagogue, its lactogenic properties are only beginning to be studied and understood. In 2011, Chinese researchers were able to establish a link between papaya consumption and improved breastfeeding rates, but the reason why papaya can increase milk supply is still unknown.[34]

Holy Basil and Lemon Basil

The leaves of the holy or sacred basil plant as well as the leaves of the lemon basil plant are both used to improve milk production in Thailand.[35] Holy and lemon basil look similar to traditional sweet basil commonly found in the United States; however, they have a more aromatic scent and deeper flavor.

Fennel

Fennel is often used as an adjunct herb, meaning that it's used in conjunction with another lactogenic food such as barley or fenugreek. The fennel seed is more often used as a galactagogue than the mature plant; however, both the seed and the mature plant contain phytoestrogens that are believed to help increase milk production.[36]

POTENTIAL LACTOGENIC FOODS AND HERBS

The list of traditional herbs and foods used throughout mammalian history to help improve milk production is vast and grows daily.

As our collective wisdom grows and we begin to learn the ancient secrets that cultures around the world have known for thousands of years, new purported galactagogues also appear. While the following foods haven't been proven to be lactogenic in a clinical setting and/or don't have enough consistent anecdotal or historical evidence about their efficacy, they're sometimes considered lactogenic:

Dill

Apricots

Asparagus

Garlic

Red beets

Sesame seeds

Poppy seeds

Caraway seeds

Anise seeds

Coriander seeds

In some cultures, mothers will consume their placenta either cooked or encapsulated in pill form to help increase milk supply, although there is no clinical evidence that this is the case.

SUPERFOODS TO HELP YOU BREASTFEED

As a breastfeeding mother, you're a milk-making machine twenty-four hours a day! There isn't a moment in the day that your body isn't actively making milk for your little one. Many breastfeeding mothers report feeling constantly hungry, and this hunger comes from the amount of calories that your body uses making each ounce of milk. Fueling your body with nutrient-dense foods that help replenish it with everything it needs is vital. While the breastfeeding superfoods in this section have not been clinically proven to be lactogenic, many have been used for centuries all around the world to nourish nursing mothers and contain a nutrient-rich mix of healthy fats, vitamins, minerals, phytonutrients, and antioxidants that are ideal for the breastfeeding mother.

Avocados

Avocados are a nutritional powerhouse for nursing moms. A common complaint of nursing mothers is that they are often very hungry due to the increased caloric demands of nursing and have very little time to prep and eat meals. Avocados are nearly 80 percent fat and help maintain a feeling of fullness in addition to providing your body with heart-healthy fats. Avocados are also a good source of B vitamins, vitamin K, folate, potassium, vitamin C, and vitamin E.

Nuts

Another powerhouse of nutrition, nuts are high in essential minerals such as iron, calcium, and zinc as well as vitamin K and B vitamins. They are also a healthy source of essential fatty acids and protein. Beyond their phenomenal nutritional makeup, nuts are also regarded as lactogenic foods in many parts of the world. While there's little clinical evidence to substantiate the use of nuts as a galactagogue, they have been used in traditional ayurvedic medicine for generations, especially almonds, which are not only written about extensively in ayurvedic literature but are one of the most widely used lactogenic foods in the world.[37]

Beans and Legumes

Beans and legumes are good sources of protein, vitamins, minerals, and phytoestrogens. Chickpeas have been used as a galactagogue since the time of ancient Egypt and are a staple food in North African, Middle Eastern, and Mediterranean cuisine, making them one of the most highly accessible galactagogues.[38] Although chickpeas are the most traditionally used lactogenic legume, there's no need to limit yourself to one type of bean or legume for its lactogenic properties. For instance, soybeans have the highest phytoestrogen content of all beans. Eating a variety of beans and legumes is good not only for your general health, but also for helping to ensure that you have a healthy milk supply.

Mushrooms

Mushrooms aren't typically regarded as lactogenic foods, but certain types of mushrooms are good sources of the polysaccharide beta-glucan, thought to be the principle lactogenic agent responsible for the galactagogue properties of both barley and oats.[39] Because barley and oats have proven lactogenic power, it's not a stretch to deduce that other foods high in beta-glucans such as mushrooms would have the same lactogenic effects. In my own clinical practice, I've found that women who increase their intake of beta-glucan rich foods such as oats,

barley, certain types of mushrooms, yeast, and algae/seaweed have seen an increase in milk production. Reishi, shiitake, maitake, shimeji, and oyster mushrooms have the highest beta-glucan content in the mushroom family.

Green Leafy Vegetables

In Thailand, a mother's first line of defense against low milk supply is the consumption of vegetables.[40] While there's no current published research on the lactogenic properties of green leafy vegetables, consuming more vegetables will only benefit your health while also establishing good eating habits for your baby to follow when she begins consuming solids around six months of age. Green leafy vegetables contain phytoestrogens, which have been shown to have a positive effect on milk production. This may be the key to understanding their lactogenic power.[41] Many mothers worry that consuming green leafy vegetables such as broccoli or cabbage will increase gassiness and fussiness in their infant. However, this is not true: The carbohydrate portion of these vegetables, which is what can cause gas, cannot transfer into the breast milk.

Red and Orange Root Vegetables

While red and orange vegetables have yet to be studied specifically for their galactagogue properties, they have been used as lactogenic foods in many cultures around the world for hundreds of years. Red and orange root vegetables such as carrots and yams have also been used for generations in the traditional Chinese *zuo yuezi* diet (*zuo yuezi* means "sit the month" and is a time of resting for new mothers) with the belief that they not only nourish the mother but help her nourish the child by increasing the quality and quantity of her breast milk.[42] Any lactogenic properties that red and orange root vegetables might have are likely similar to those of green leafy vegetables. The phytoestrogens in these plants in addition to their high-nutrient density may play a role in improving breast milk.

Seeds

Seeds are a nutritional gift! They are the very beginning of life for every plant on earth. They provide a concentrated source of all the nutrients found in the mature plant as well as the nutrients needed to grow the tiny seed into a beautiful blooming plant. Seeds are high in protein and essential minerals such as iron, zinc, and calcium, as well as healthy fats. Like nuts, seeds are not clinically proven to have lactogenic properties, but they have been used for centuries to help breastfeeding mothers thanks to their high vitamin and mineral content. Every seed has its unique nutritional makeup, so choose a variety including sunflower seeds, pumpkin seeds, and sesame seeds.

CHIA SEEDS

While chia seeds might seem like a new phenomenon, they have been widely consumed for centuries and were a staple food of the Aztecs and Mayans. Chia seeds are not only a rich source of fiber, protein, calcium, and magnesium but also have a high omega-3 fatty acid content. Due to their high fiber and protein content as well as their favorable fatty acid concentration, chia seeds help you feel more satisfied and fuller longer after a meal. Chia oil is also an excellent source of omega-3 fatty acids and has a neutral and pleasant flavor.

HEMP SEEDS

Like chia seeds, hemp seeds have found their way onto this superfood list due to their high content of omega-3 fatty acids and healthy nutrient composition. Hemp seeds have a favorable omega-3 to omega-6 ratio of 3:1 (see page 97 for more about this important number) and are a complete protein, meaning they contain all of the essential amino acids needed by the human body in perfect proportions. While hemp seeds are high in many vitamins and minerals, they are especially high in iron and zinc, which are important for infant growth and maternal health.

FLAXSEEDS

Flaxseeds are an excellent source of protein, fiber, and omega-3 fatty acids, but in order to unlock their benefits, they must be ground—whole flaxseeds can't be digested in the body and are excreted unchanged. Flax oil is also an excellent source of omega-3 fatty acids and has a sweet and light taste that pairs well with veggies and blends seamlessly into smoothies. The studied health benefits of flaxseeds are far-reaching, from weight loss and blood glucose control to reduced risk of certain types of cancers, cardiovascular disease, and inflammation.

Turmeric

Although turmeric is used throughout the world by breastfeeding mothers as a galactagogue, there's no clinical evidence to support that the herb has any effect on the volume of breast milk a mother produces. However, the anti-inflammatory properties of turmeric have been demonstrated in clinical studies to be important to the health and well-being of breastfeeding mothers for the prevention and treatment of mastitis as well as to ease the symptoms associated with breast engorgement (see pages 40 and 17 for more on these conditions). In several communities throughout Asia, turmeric is also believed to help boost the immune system of not only mom but baby, to ward off coughs and colds.[43]

Ashwagandha

Ashwagandha is an herb used traditionally in ayurvedic medicine that goes by many other names, including Indian ginseng and winter cherry. Ashwagandha is considered a multipurpose herb that works on several body systems at once, including the neurologic, immune, endocrine, and reproductive systems. Though it hasn't been shown to have any specific lactogenic properties, it's a godsend to breastfeeding mothers who are experiencing stress. In clinical studies, 300 mg twice a day of ashwagandha extract significantly reduced stress in study participants. Not only did the participants who received ashwagandha feel a greater relief of their overall stress and an increase in their quality of life, but their cortisol levels were significantly lower.[44] Ashwagandha also seems to have an effect on endurance and energy, although the reasons for this are still unknown.[45] Ashwagandha is a well-studied herb with more than sixty research articles available on its use for a variety of different disease processes, although the exact mechanism by which it works is still unknown.[46] When you think of the many ways that stress affects every system in your body, it's easy to see how ashwagandha's effect on stress hormones can influence the rest of the body as well.

Fermented Foods

Fermented foods, from pickles to miso soup, contain a stockpile of highly digestible forms of macro- and micronutrients as well as phytonutrients. Better yet, they provide a broad spectrum of probiotics, which are important to maintaining a healthy GI tract. Although our intestines are the first thing many people think of when they think of the GI tract, the GI tract is the entire route from the mouth to the anus. This includes the mouth, esophagus, stomach, small intestines, and large intestines. Your digestive tract is approximately thirty feet long! That is a lot of real estate to keep healthy and functioning well.

Probiotics are a relatively new addition to our discussion on health and wellness in the United States, where we typically find the broadest-spectrum probiotics available in supplement form; however, probiotic-rich foods are a central component in diets around the world. The earliest records of probiotic-rich foods date back to 6000 BCE. In Korea, kimchi has been an integral part of daily nutrition since 57 BCE. Other common foods you might have heard of that are rich in probiotics are sauerkraut, pickled vegetables, yogurt, kombucha, kefir, natto, miso, tempeh, fermented tofu, and raw apple cider vinegar. But the list of fermented foods goes far beyond that and even includes fermented beers and wines. Western science is just now catching up with ancient traditional wisdom from around the world.

To our present knowledge, probiotics don't readily transfer from the mother's diet into her breast milk; however, a healthy GI tract is incredibly important to the overall health of not only breastfeeding mothers but all humans. More studies are emerging on the positive effects probiotics have on controlling diet-induced obesity, yeast in the body (candidiasis), type 2 diabetes, inflammation, metabolic function, cancers, vaginal infections, *H. pylori*, heart disease (high cholesterol, hypertension, and hyperlipidemia), eczema, liver disease, food allergies, GI disorders (irritable bowel disease, irritable bowel syndrome, and diarrhea), and overall immunity.[47]

Probiotics have also been shown to improve the nutritional value of foods through a variety of mechanisms, including freeing amino acids and improving the synthesis of vitamins.[48]

ANTILACTOGENIC FOODS, HERBS, AND MEDICATIONS

The phytochemicals and phytonutrients in many plants have the ability to not only nourish your body but also increase the quality and quantity of your milk supply. Similarly, there are some medications that have the side effect of increasing milk supply through increased serum prolactin levels. However, not all foods and herbs increase milk supply. In fact, some plants, herbs, and medications can decrease milk supply. Some, like alcohol or parsley, will slowly decrease milk supply, while others, like pseudoephedrine, will dramatically stop the production of milk within hours of the first dose. In this section, you'll learn all about the food, herbs, and medications that can decrease your milk supply.

Alcohol

For many years, health care providers recommended that mothers enjoy a beer before nursing to help with the milk ejection reflex, offer relaxation, boost milk supply, and improve milk quality. However, this advice was a bit misguided. While alcohol certainly has the ability to help one relax, it does so by acting as a depressant of the central nervous system. It also blocks the release of oxytocin, which results in a decrease of circulating oxytocin and a decrease in the amount of letdowns a mother will have in each nursing session.[49] In studies, after mothers consumed a modest amount of alcohol, infants initially seemed to suck more frequently. However, pre- and post-feed weights revealed that infants who are fed milk by mothers who have consumed alcohol tend to take in less milk than mothers who were consuming a nonalcoholic placebo. The reason behind this is not yet understood, although it has been noted that alcohol can change the taste and odor of human milk.[50] Mothers have reported that their breasts feel much fuller after drinking alcohol; however, we now know the full feeling is the result of inefficient milk transfer to the infant due to alcohol consumption by the breastfeeding mother. It turns out that the myth that alcohol improves milk supply is rooted in the fact that many types of beer used to contain therapeutic levels of barley or barley malt, which are known galactagogues. However, modern beer-making results in subtherapeutic levels of barley or oats.

The recommendation still stands that four ounces of wine, one ounce of hard liquor, or eight ounces of beer will not have any appreciable negative impact on your infant, your milk supply, or your infant's ability to nurse. Any amounts beyond this should be avoided. (See page 20 for information about "pumping and dumping," which is usually unnecessary.)

While the occasional alcoholic beverage won't negatively impact your milk supply, in the long term, chronic alcohol consumption will negatively impact your milk quality and milk volume. Additionally, after a night of heavy drinking, you'll notice that your milk supply rapidly declines. Some women are able to recover quickly from this rapid decline, usually within twenty-four to forty-eight hours. For other women, frequent pumping in addition to galactagogues will be needed to build back a healthy milk supply that will meet the nutritional needs of your baby.

Sage, Parsley, Peppermint, and Menthol

Many herbs are naturally lactogenic foods that can provide you with the boost in breast milk production you're looking for. However, not all herbs are created equal. Sage, parsley, peppermint, and menthol have all been noted to decrease milk supply in women who consume large quantities of each. There are no formal studies that look at the exact quantity needed for each herb to make a negative impact on breastfeeding; however, anecdotal evidence has shown that these herbs can and do decrease milk supply. You don't need to worry about avoiding each of these herbs altogether, but be mindful of dishes that contain large amounts. For instance, sage is a popular herb used around on Thanksgiving, parsley is found in large quantities in dishes like tabbouleh, and peppermint is often found in teas, gums, and candies.

Chasteberry

Chasteberry, the dried fruit of the chaste tree, is native to the Mediterranean. It has long been used for a variety of reproductive issues including symptoms related to PMS, endometriosis, and menopause. Chasteberry has also traditionally been used to help breastfeeding mothers who are experiencing engorgement or any other type of painful swelling of the breast. However, chasteberry exerts its therapeutic effects by acting directly on the pituitary gland and inhibits the secretion of prolactin.[51] When prolactin levels are reduced in a breastfeeding mother, milk supply typically reduces with it. Therefore, it isn't recommended that breastfeeding mothers take chasteberry supplements for the duration of lactation. If you're looking for an herb to help ease the inflammation associated with engorgement, turmeric (page 117) is a well-studied option that doesn't have a negative effect on milk supply.

Pseudoephedrine, Methergine, and Bromocriptine

Some medicines adversely affect breastfeeding. Pseudoephedrine (the active ingredient in Sudafed and similar cold medications), Methergine (often used to treat severe uterine bleeding after childbirth), and bromocriptine (brand names Parlodel or Cycloset, used for a variety of issues) have been shown to have a negative effect on milk supply.[52] If your supply has dropped, and you realize you've taken one of the medications listed here, ask your doctor about an alternative treatment for your cold or health ailment. Increased breastfeeding, supplementation with lactogenic herbs and foods, and possibly additional pumping will help you build up your milk production again.

OTHER FOODS TO AVOID

Unsafely Prepared Foods

Passing on harmful pathogens like those involved in food poisoning to your baby via breast milk is very rare, but it's still important to always practice safe food-handling procedures. At the age of six months, your little one, who is still getting 100 percent of her nutrients from breast milk, will transition to getting about 85 percent from breast milk and 15 percent from complementary foods by the end of her first year of life. So starting good food-safety habits now is important. Always wash your hands and any surface you'll

be preparing food on thoroughly before cooking. Additionally, make sure to keep cross-contamination to a minimum. Cut meats and vegetables with different knives and be sure to clean your cutting board thoroughly when switching from cutting meats to vegetables (or just use a separate cutting board for each). Finally, make sure your food is cooked through completely and at a safe temperature to prevent proliferation of food-borne illnesses.

Caffeine

Many mothers are excited to finally get back to their morning latte routine after giving birth. Unfortunately, more often than not, moms quickly find out that reintroducing caffeine into their diet too soon can lead to a fussy and overtired infant. This is because caffeine is a stimulant that readily passes into breast milk. While the half-life of caffeine in adults is approximately 4.9 hours, the half-life of caffeine in infants can be as high as 97.5 hours (four or more days)![53]

The older the infant is, the better she will tolerate caffeine. Studies have shown that by three to six months of age, most infants' sleep wasn't adversely affected by maternal caffeine consumption.[54] Based on the clinical evidence available, I advise my patients to wait until their infant is at least three months old to reintroduce caffeine into their diet and then watch their baby for any signs of discomfort or restlessness. For moms who work outside the home, I suggest that you always label any pumped milk that you have expressed after consuming caffeine to ensure that the infant is not given this milk right before naptime or bedtime. While coffee, tea, chocolate, and soda are obvious sources of caffeine, there are also significant amounts of caffeine in coffee- and chocolate-flavored foods and beverages. Even decaffeinated coffee has some caffeine in it, so keep this in mind if your baby is especially sensitive to it.

High-Mercury Fish

When cooked in a healthy manner (such as baking or broiling), fish can be a nutrient-rich component of your diet. However, due to a wide array of factors, most fish and other seafood also contain unhealthy chemicals, particularly mercury. Mercury is an element found in the Earth's crust that is typically only released in unhealthy quantities during events like a volcanic eruption. Unfortunately, mining, waste incineration, and other industrial processes release unsafe quantities of mercury into the environment. In the body, mercury can accumulate and quickly rise to dangerous levels. High levels of mercury principally affect the central nervous system, causing neurological defects.[55] For this reason, the US Food and Drug Administration (FDA), Environmental Protection Agency (EPA), and WHO have all cautioned against the consumption of high-mercury foods for pregnant women, nursing mothers, and children. As mercury is considered by the WHO to be one of the top ten chemicals of major public health concern, there are also specific guidelines set forth by the EPA for healthy adults based on weight and gender.[56] In general, no more than two to three servings (a maximum of twelve ounces) of low-mercury fish should be eaten in a week.

Fish that tend to contain low levels of mercury include salmon, flounder, tilapia, trout, pollock, and catfish. (It should be noted, however, that all these fish still do contain mercury, just in lower levels.) Meanwhile, tuna, shark, swordfish, mackerel, and tilefish all tend to have higher levels of mercury and should be avoided. On a lighter note, for moms who have been waiting patiently for forty weeks to eat sushi, you can rest assured that sushi not containing high-mercury fish is considered safe for breastfeeding mothers due to the fact that the *Listeria* bacteria, which can be found in undercooked foods, is not transmitted readily through breast milk.

FREQUENTLY ASKED QUESTIONS

ARE THERE ANY MEDICATIONS THAT HAVE BEEN SHOWN TO IMPROVE MILK SUPPLY?

There are, but they are of limited availability, and none have been approved by the FDA to treat low milk supply. Because prolactin works with other hormones, dopamine-antagonist drugs such as domperidone and metoclopramide have very favorable clinical evidence of working to increase a mother's milk supply by increasing her prolactin levels.[1] In addition, a number of psychoactive drugs (such as phenothiazines) have been used both in clinical practice and in a worldwide clinical study and were shown to increase prolactin levels in breastfeeding mothers. In extreme cases, oversupply of milk resulted from their use.

However, of these medications, the only one that is currently available in the United States is metoclopramide—brand name Reglan—which is generally prescribed for gastroesophageal reflux disease (GERD). Based on current clinical studies and guidelines, an increased milk supply is typically seen when women take 10 to 15 mg of metoclopramide three to four times a day for four to fourteen days.[2] While it doesn't appear that metoclopramide transfers to the infant via breast milk, the drug can pose serious side effects for the breastfeeding mother,[3] including seizures and depression. Since new mothers are already at a higher risk of depression, metoclopramide might not be a good choice for many breastfeeding mothers.

SHOULD I CONTINUE TO TAKE VITAMINS AND SUPPLEMENTS?

Many health care practitioners recommend that breastfeeding mothers continue to take prenatal vitamins; however, the nutrient needs of a pregnant woman are very different from those of a breastfeeding woman. Prenatal and multivitamins should only be used on a case-by-case basis after your nutrition status has been evaluated by a dietitian or other qualified health care professional. Taking synthetic vitamins in excess of your individual needs can cause more harm than good for your short- and long-term health.[4] Additionally, supplementation with synthetic vitamins, minerals, and antioxidants has not been shown to lower disease risk, improve disease outcomes, or improve overall health.[5] While it can be alluring to look at the side of a vitamin bottle and see that you've had 100 percent or more of your daily nutrient needs met by taking a pill, the fact is that synthetic vitamins are absorbed poorly by the body (with the exception of folic acid). The majority of vitamins and minerals taken in supplement form are either excreted in your urine or stored in your body at levels that can be detrimental to your health. Many vitamins have a tolerable upper intake level, and some even have toxicity levels. And while reaching toxicity levels of a vitamin or mineral is typically quite hard to do by eating foods, it's much easier to do with supplement usage, even for those that claim to be made directly from fruits and vegetables.

Chances are that if you're eating a healthy, well-balanced diet, then you're getting all the nutrients you need. Our bodies are more flexible than we give them credit for, and they don't require that we eat perfectly every meal and every day to obtain the nutrients we need for health and wellness. Our bodies are designed to go through periods when certain vitamins and minerals are plentiful and periods when they are not. If you're concerned about your macro- or micronutrient intake, make an appointment to see a registered dietitian who specializes in maternal nutrition to evaluate your diet and nutrition status.

CAN DIET CAUSE A FUSSY BABY?

A common myth about breastfeeding and nutrition is that there are certain foods a mother can eat that make an infant gassy or fussy. Like most myths or urban legends, it is based on a bit of truth. Some infants do have allergies or intolerances to certain foods (usually protein based) that can have painful and unpleasant side effects. While food allergies such as a casein allergy can be attributed to GI upset and distress, other foods like broccoli, beans, and cabbage do not pass readily into breast milk and, therefore, do not cause fussiness in infants. Breast milk is made from blood, which means that compounds that travel through the blood, such as iron from supplements, vitamins and minerals, proteins, and glucose, can travel into breast milk. But problems in the intestines stay isolated to the intestines and don't pass into breast milk. This is why the intestinal upset that typically follows food poisoning doesn't transfer to your baby.

There are myriad reasons for a fussy infant. Being born, in and of itself, is quite a big adjustment! The sudden change from a warm, dark, wet, and quiet environment to a loud, dry, and bright environment where the temperature is constantly changing is a jarring one, and one that an infant doesn't adjust to overnight. Additionally, growth spurts, being tired or overtired, and experiencing even the smallest separation from his primary caregiver can cause fussiness in an infant. Some mothers will tell you that when that they removed broccoli from their diet, their infants became less fussy. Typically, these kind of associations are coincidences. In many cases, by the time moms begin eliminating foods from their diets, the causes of their infants' fussiness have already passed.

HOW DO I KNOW IF MY BABY HAS A FOOD ALLERGY?

Food allergies seem all too common these days, from peanut-free schools to the boom in dairy-free and gluten-free food options in not only health food but conventional grocery stores and restaurants. It can seem, at times, that nearly everyone has a food allergy or knows someone who does. However, the fact is that food allergies are actually quite rare and typically overreported. Current statistics show that approximately 5 percent of children and 3 percent of adults have food allergies. This data comes from self-reported information, meaning that parents are surveyed and asked, "During the past twelve months, has your child had any kind of food or digestive allergy?"[6] This means that the current data we have on allergy prevalence for infants and children are based purely on parental perception. It has been well documented that the term *allergy* means different things to different people, with a large divide between what is medically considered an allergy and what the average person considers an allergy.[7] The medical definition of an allergic reaction is an IgE-mediated response to an allergen, usually a food protein. Simply put, this means that the body is launching an immune-based response to a normal food item—one's body is overreacting to a normally harmless food. Food allergies are very different from food sensitivities or intolerances, which don't involve the immune system. The rate of perception of food allergies is estimated to be about four times higher than the actual true prevalence of food allergies.[8]

To truly identify if an individual has an immune-mediated food allergy, a skin test is one of the most reliable methods. The most reliable method of food allergy identification is a food challenge in which the child is exposed to an allergen in a controlled setting, such as an allergist's office, and response to the allergen is noted. However, it might prove difficult to identify digestive or delayed responses to an allergen via a food challenge, as they can take four to twelve hours to manifest. Blood tests in general are often unreliable and not the best assessment tool for food allergens.[9]

Assessing whether or not an infant is allergic to a food can often be a difficult task. Blood and skin tests are very intrusive to tiny little bodies and aren't recommended. Therefore, we are left to make an educated guess based on symptoms and the current scientific evidence as to what type of allergy an infant might have, if any, and how to help a mother eliminate the offending foods from her diet in order to continue breastfeeding.

The principle protein in cow's milk, casein, is often the first place we look when it comes to perceived allergies in infants. Human milk is high in another form of milk protein called whey. Whey is easily digested by humans. However, beta-casein, which is present in cow's milk but not in human milk, is very difficult for humans to digest, as it's a foreign protein to our bodies. Beta-casein passes easily into the breast milk and can cause digestive upset in infants, ranging from gassiness, fussiness, and colic symptoms to projectile vomiting. It's important to note that this adverse reaction to cow's milk isn't based on the lactose content of cow's milk, and reducing or eliminating lactose from your diet won't have any effect on your baby's symptoms. Human milk is actually higher in lactose than cow's milk, and lactose intolerance in infancy is not only incredibly rare but also life-threatening! Instead, if an infant is showing signs of a casein intolerance or allergy, a mother will need to eliminate all products containing casein from her diet, including all dairy. Many mothers are advised against drinking cow's milk and nursing, out of concern for the gut health of the growing infant. While this blanket statement isn't true for all babies, it's true for many. Casein takes up to four weeks to completely clear the body, which is why many practitioners do recommend that casein be removed from the diet immediately if an infant shows symptoms of casein intolerance or allergy.

If a dairy elimination diet doesn't resolve your infant's symptoms, then there might be another food that's causing your little one discomfort. The top food allergens for children tend to be milk, eggs, and soy.[10] Tackling an elimination diet can be daunting on your own while also trying to balance the demands of motherhood. It's recommended that you work with a registered dietitian well versed in breastfeeding on a safe elimination diet that ensures you're continuing to get all the nutrients you need to nourish yourself and your infant.

CAN MY DIET AFFECT THE NUTRIENT CONTENT OR QUALITY OF MY MILK?

In general, your diet can't affect the quality of your breast milk. While eating a well-balanced diet is the best option to maintain your own health, it does not have a major impact on the quality of your breast milk. If your diet is severely nutrient and calorie deficient, the quantity of your milk will decrease, but not the quality, meaning that your body will choose to make a smaller amount of good-quality milk than a large amount of subpar milk. (In cases of starvation, however, the body will typically opt to stop making milk altogether, as it no longer has the available calories to pull from you to make milk.)

It's important that you continue to nourish yourself in the most optimal way possible so you can continue to nourish your baby in the most optimal way possible, and many of the foods and herbs I've listed to boost your breast milk not only will make sure you have a healthy supply but are also full of the nutrients your baby will be using. But rest assured, that brownie you had earlier today didn't negatively affect the quality of your milk.

HOW DO I CHOOSE THE LACTOGENIC FOODS THAT ARE RIGHT FOR ME?

Looking at the list of lactogenic herbs, foods, and medications available to you, it can be overwhelming to know where to begin. In my research for this book, the one thing that presented itself time and time again when looking at traditional breastfeeding diets all around the world is that healthy, whole foods that are rich in nutrients and phytonutrients were staples in every diet. Even the herbs that have been traditionally used for generations all tend to have positive effects on a variety of health matters, including chronic disease such as diabetes, cardiovascular disease, cancers, and infertility.

As a general rule, if you're currently not making enough milk to meet your infant's nutrient needs, a lactogenic herb such as moringa, fenugreek, milk thistle, or shatavari combined with lactogenic foods like oats, barley, and whole grains is a great place to start. If you're trying to protect your milk supply, then incorporating lactogenic foods such as papaya, whole grains, fennel, and oats in your diet is a great choice.

ARE LACTOGENIC FOODS AND GALACTAGOGUES SAFE FOR MY FAMILY TO EAT?

One thing that most lactogenic foods and herbs have in common is that they are used around the world for far more than just their milk-making properties. These foods are typically incredibly nutrient-dense, plant-based foods that aren't only appropriate for your entire family but extraordinarily beneficial to the short- and long-term health of your entire family! I am a big proponent of only having to make a single meal for your whole family, and each recipe in this book is a healthy addition to your family's menu not only while you're breastfeeding but throughout every stage of life.

IS IT OK TO TAKE MORE THAN ONE GALACTAGOGUE AT A TIME?

Most mothers come into my office already on their own cocktail of lactogenic herbs or foods that they read about online or were told to take by a friend. Many have started taking these galactagogues far before it was necessary and now have an oversupply of milk, while others are taking an herb incorrectly or at a dose in which benefits won't be seen. Taking every lactogenic herb and food at once isn't necessary to rebuild a healthy milk supply—ingesting multiple herbs that increase prolactin levels at the same time is typically no more effective than taking one or two.

Also, the type of galactagogue that you use is dependent upon the cause of your low milk supply. While this book will give you a good base of knowledge, if you're experiencing low milk supply and none of the solutions in Chapter 6 work, you should see an International Board Certified Lactation Consultant who can assess your medical history and breastfeeding challenges and make the best choice for you and your situation. For a mother who initially made enough milk but now finds herself overstressed and overtired due to outside influences, an herb such as fenugreek might not be effective, but a relaxing and calming herb such as ashwagandha or lemon balm might be. For a mother who is trying to exclusively pump for a premature infant in the NICU, a combination of beta-glucan-rich foods and an herb such as moringa would be a good option to increase prolactin levels. There is no one-size-fits-all approach, and what worked well for a friend or family member might not work well for you.

HOW MUCH WATER SHOULD I BE DRINKING?

Physicians, midwives, nurses, and lactation consultants will all tell you to stay well hydrated while nursing. However, hydration is a relatively understudied area of lactation with only a small handful of studies exploring the topic. What we do know is that hydration is important to all humans, lactating or not. It's especially essential for a healthy pregnancy, as it maintains the integrity of amniotic fluid.[11] Many breastfeeding mothers report feeling thirstier either directly before or after a nursing session. While the actual hydration needs of a breastfeeding mother are still unknown, studies have shown that many lactating mothers consume up to 16 percent more fluids in a day than their nonbreastfeeding counterparts.[12] It's important to note that moderate dehydration does not appear to negatively affect milk production, but the effects of chronic dehydration haven't been adequately measured in the breastfeeding mother. It's a good rule of thumb for everyone to stay well hydrated and drink somewhere between six and ten eight-ounce cups of water a day (48 to 80 ounces total) for general health.

PART FOUR

The
Recipes

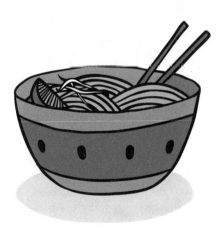

A NOTE ABOUT THE RECIPES

Recipes for lactation cookies, "leaky lemonade," and breastfeeding brownies are constantly circulating on social media and blogs. As tempting as it is to make mass quantities of pastries and desserts in the name of boosting your breast milk supply, lactogenic recipes are not confined to sweets. In fact, wholesome meals for your entire family can be built on milk-making foods and herbs.

In addition to adding a few new milk-making recipes to your repertoire, lactogenic foods and herbs are all plant based, which means they are also an excellent way of adding more fruits and vegetables to your growing family's diet. Every recipe in this section is infused with milk-making foods or breast-feeding superfoods. You'll note that above each recipe, the designation "Milk Makers" and/or "Superfoods" shows quickly what ingredients in the dish you are about to prepare are ideal for you as a breastfeeding mother.

Additionally, each recipe contains nutrition information so you can get a quick glimpse at the nutrient content of each recipe. Please refer to the nutrient needs for breastfeeding mothers on page 103 to determine how much of a nutrient you need in a day. When looking at nutrition facts, it is important to remember that you do not need to get all your nutrients from one dish; in fact, that is nearly impossible to do—and not the way our bodies were made to digest and absorb nutrients. Instead, a well-balanced daily meal plan will include foods that have a variety of nutrients in them so that by the end of the day you have reached your nutrient goals.

You'll also see that some recipes have "Rich in . . ." below the nutrition facts information. Dishes that are rich in a nutrient contain at least 10 percent of that nutrient. In recipes that call for milk, plain hemp milk (page 139) has been used for the nutritional reference unless otherwise noted.

At every turn, I have made a conscious effort to include the most nutrient-dense foods in recipes as possible, from using ground chia seed as a binder for added omega-3 fatty acids, to heart-healthy nonhydrogenated oils such as those found in Earth Balance margarine. But don't worry, there is still a little good old all-purpose flour here and there—it's all about balance, after all!

One milk-making ingredient you will see referenced quite a bit, especially in baked goods and breakfast foods, is oat flour. You can purchase oat flour, but it is very simple, and much less expensive, to make at home. To make oat flour, simply process 2 cups (80 g) rolled oats in a food processor or even a blender until you have a fine flour. This should take anywhere from 30 to 60 seconds, sometimes a little longer depending on the quality of your food processor or blender. This will give you about 2 cups of oat flour, and you'll still have plenty of leftover whole rolled oats to make Oatmeal Milk-In Cookies (page 212) or Hemp Seed Oatmeal (page 156).

MILK-MAKIN' MILKS

Plant-based milks are a quick and easy way to give your recipes a nutrient boost while also powering them with more milk-making and enriching components like beta-glucan, omega-3 essential fatty acids, and protein. While the task of making your own milk might seem exhausting, it typically only takes about 5 minutes to gather your ingredients, blend, and serve. Any of the unflavored milks in this section can be used for recipes throughout this book or for any recipe that calls for milk.

Oat Milk

MAKES 4 CUPS (960 ML)
MILK MAKER: oats

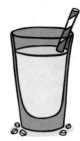

3½ cups (840 ml) filtered water
1 cup (80 g) rolled oats
2 tablespoons maple syrup or agave nectar
1 teaspoon vanilla extract

1. Pour 2 cups (480 ml) of the water, the oats, maple syrup, and vanilla into a high-speed blender (see Note) and blend on high until smooth. While the blender is running, add the remaining 1½ cups (360 ml) water and blend until combined.

2. Refrigerate until chilled. Oat milk can be stored in an airtight container in the refrigerator for 2 to 3 days. Shake thoroughly before using.

NOTE: If not using a high-speed blender, you will need to strain your milk. To strain the oat milk, pour it through a nut milk bag (or cheesecloth) into a pitcher or bowl. Use your hands to squeeze the milk out of your nut milk bag. Once you have squeezed out all the milk, you can discard the oat pulp.

PER SERVING (1 CUP/240 ML) Calories: 190; total fat: 2.5 g; saturated fat: 0 g; cholesterol: 0 mg/dl; sodium: 10 mg; total carbohydrate: 36 g; dietary fiber: 4 g; sugar: 11 g; protein: 7 g; vitamin A: 0 mcg; vitamin C: 0 mg; calcium: 40 mg; iron: 1.8 mg
Rich in iron, thiamin, riboflavin, phosphorus, magnesium, zinc, copper, and manganese

Barley Milk

MAKES 4 CUPS (960 ML)
MILK MAKER: barley

1 cup (80 g) barley flakes
3½ cups (840 ml) filtered water

3 tablespoons maple syrup or agave nectar

1. Pour the barley, 2 cups (480 ml) of the water, and maple syrup into a high-speed blender (see Note) and blend on high until smooth. While the blender is running, add the remaining 1½ cups (360 ml) water and blend until combined.

2. Refrigerate until chilled. Barley milk can be stored in an airtight container in the refrigerator for 2 to 3 days. Shake thoroughly before using.

> **NOTE:** If not using a high-speed blender, you will need to strain your milk. To strain the barley milk, pour it through a nut milk bag (or cheesecloth) into a pitcher or bowl. Use your hands to squeeze the milk out of your nut milk bag. Once you have squeezed out all the milk, you can discard the barley pulp.

PER SERVING (1 CUP/240 ML) Calories: 120; total fat: 0.5 g; saturated fat: 0 g; cholesterol: 0 mg/dl; sodium: 5 mg; total carbohydrate: 26 g; dietary fiber: 3 g; sugar: 10 g; protein: 3 g; vitamin A: 0 mcg; vitamin C: 0 mg; calcium: 20 mg; iron: 1 mg
Rich in riboflavin and manganese

Sesame Milk

MAKES 5½ CUPS (1.3 L)
SUPERFOODS: sesame seeds, hemp oil

4 cups (960 ml) filtered water
1 cup (145 g) sesame seeds

3 tablespoons maple syrup
1 tablespoon hemp oil

1. Pour 2 cups (480 ml) of the water, the sesame seeds, and maple syrup into a high-speed blender (see Note) and blend on high until smooth. While the blender is running, add the remaining 2 cups (480 ml) water and the hemp oil, and blend until combined.

2. Refrigerate until chilled. Sesame milk can be stored in an airtight container in the refrigerator for 2 to 3 days. Shake thoroughly before using.

> **NOTE:** If not using a high-speed blender, you will need to strain your milk. To strain the sesame milk, pour it through a nut milk bag (or cheesecloth) into a pitcher or bowl. Use your hands to squeeze the milk out of your nut milk bag. Once you have squeezed out all the milk, you can discard the sesame seed pulp.

PER SERVING (1 CUP/240 ML) Calories: 200; total fat: 15 g; saturated fat: 2 g; cholesterol: 0 mg/dl; sodium: 10 mg; total carbohydrate: 13 g; dietary fiber: 3 g; sugar: 7 g; protein: 5 g; vitamin A: 0 mcg; vitamin C: 0 mg; calcium: 250 mg; iron: 3.6 mg
Rich in calcium, iron, thiamin, riboflavin, vitamin B6, phosphorus, magnesium, zinc, selenium, copper, and manganese

Hemp Milk

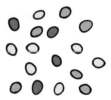

MAKES 4½ CUPS (1 L)
SUPERFOOD: hemp seeds

3½ cups (840 ml) filtered water

½ cup (80 g) organic raw, shelled hemp seeds

2 to 3 tablespoons maple syrup or agave nectar

1 teaspoon soy or sunflower lecithin, optional

1. Pour 2 cups (480 ml) of the filtered water and the hemp seeds into a high-speed blender and blend until smooth. While the blender is still running, add the remaining 1½ cups (360 ml) water, the maple syrup to taste, and lecithin, if using.

RECIPE CONTINUES →

2. Refrigerate until chilled. Hemp milk can be stored in an airtight container in the refrigerator for 3 to 4 days.

PER SERVING (1 CUP/240 ML) Calories: 120; total fat: 8 g; saturated fat: 1 g; cholesterol: 0 mg/dl; sodium: 0 mg; total carbohydrate: 8 g; dietary fiber: 2 g; sugar: 6 g; protein: 6 g; vitamin A: 0 mcg; vitamin C: 0 mg; calcium: 20 mg; iron: 1.8 mg

Rich in iron, thiamin, riboflavin, phosphorus, magnesium, zinc, and manganese

Chocolate Malt Milk

MAKES 3¾ CUPS (890 ML)
MILK MAKER: barley
SUPERFOOD: hemp seeds

3 cups (720 ml) filtered water

½ cup (80 g) organic raw, shelled hemp seeds

3 tablespoons barley malt or maple syrup

¼ cup (45 g) sweet ground cocoa powder or 2 tablespoons unsweetened cocoa powder

½ to 1 teaspoon vanilla extract

1. Pour 2 cups (480 ml) of the filtered water and the hemp seeds into a high-speed blender and blend until smooth. While the blender is still running, add the remaining 1 cup (240 ml) water, the barley malt, cocoa powder, and vanilla to taste, and blend until smooth.

2. Refrigerate until chilled. Malt milk can be stored in an airtight container in the refrigerator for 3 to 4 days.

PER SERVING (1 CUP/240 ML) Calories: 200; total fat: 10 g; saturated fat: 1.5 g; cholesterol: 0 mg/dl; sodium: 10 mg; total carbohydrate: 19 g; dietary fiber: 4 g; sugar: 14 g; protein: 9 g; vitamin A: 0 mcg; vitamin C: 0 mg; calcium: 40 mg; iron: 3.6 mg

Rich in iron, thiamin, riboflavin, vitamin B6, phosphorus, magnesium, zinc, copper, and manganese

Almond Milk

MAKES 4½ CUPS (1 L)
SUPERFOOD: almonds

3½ cups (840 ml) filtered water
1 cup (145 g) raw almonds, soaked overnight (see Notes)
2 to 3 tablespoons maple syrup or agave nectar

OPTIONAL ADD-INS FOR CINNAMON VANILLA ALMOND MILK (SEE NOTES)
1 teaspoon vanilla extract or 1 whole vanilla bean scraped clean
¼ teaspoon ground cinnamon

1. Place all the ingredients in a high-speed blender (see Notes) and blend until smooth.

2. Refrigerate until chilled. Almond milk can be stored in an airtight container in the refrigerator for 3 to 4 days.

NOTES: It's preferable, but not mandatory, to skin the almonds after soaking them. Once the almonds have been soaked overnight, drain and rinse them. Then it's fairly easy to pop the skins off between your thumb and forefinger and discard any skins.

If you prefer plain milk, omit the cinnamon and vanilla.

If not using a high-speed blender, you will need to strain your milk. To strain the milk, pour it through a nut milk bag (or cheesecloth) into a pitcher or bowl. Use your hands to squeeze the milk out of your nut milk bag. Once you have squeezed out all the milk, you can discard the pulp.

PER SERVING (1 CUP/240 ML) Calories: 210; total fat: 16 g; saturated fat: 1 g; cholesterol: 0 mg/dl; sodium: 0 mg; total carbohydrate: 14 g; dietary fiber: 4 g; sugar: 9 g; protein: 7 g; vitamin A: 0 mcg; vitamin C: 0 mg; calcium: 100 mg; iron: 1 mg
Rich in calcium, vitamin E, riboflavin, phosphorus, magnesium, copper, and manganese

Ayurvedic Almond Milk

MAKES 2 CUPS (480 ML)
SUPERFOOD: almonds

2 cups (480 ml) filtered water

20 almonds, soaked overnight with skins removed

2 teaspoons maple syrup or agave nectar

Pinch of ground cardamom

Pinch of ground ginger

Pour the filtered water, almonds, and maple syrup into a blender and blend until smooth. Transfer to a tall glass and sprinkle with ground cardamom and ginger. Almond milk can be stored in an airtight container in the refrigerator for 3 to 4 days.

PER SERVING (1 CUP/240 ML) Calories: 90; total fat: 6 g; saturated fat: 0 g; cholesterol: 0 mg/dl; sodium: 10 mg; total carbohydrate: 7 g; dietary fiber: 2 g; sugar: 5 g; protein: 3 g; vitamin A: 0 mcg; vitamin C: 0 mg; calcium: 40 mg; iron: <1 mg
Rich in vitamin E, riboflavin, magnesium, and manganese

Cashew Milk

MAKES 4½ CUPS (1 L)
SUPERFOOD: cashews

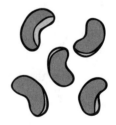

4 cups (960 ml) filtered water

1 cup (140 g) raw, unsalted cashews, soaked for 4 hours

2 tablespoons maple syrup

1. In a high-speed blender, blend 2 cups (480 ml) of the water and the cashews until smooth. While the blender is still running, add the remaining 2 cups (480 ml) water and the maple syrup.

2. Refrigerate until chilled. Cashew milk can be kept in an airtight container in the refrigerator for 3 to 4 days.

PER SERVING (1 CUP/240 ML) Calories: 180; total fat: 13 g; saturated fat: 2 g; cholesterol: 0 mg/dl; sodium: 0 mg; total carbohydrate: 15 g; dietary fiber: <1 g; sugar: 8 g; protein: 5 g; vitamin A: 0 mcg; vitamin C: 0 mg; calcium: 20 mg; iron: 1.8 mg
Rich in iron, vitamin K, phosphorus, magnesium, zinc, copper, and manganese

Pumpkin Seed Milk

MAKES 4 CUPS (960 ML)
SUPERFOOD: pumpkin seeds

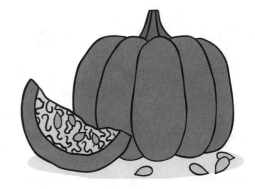

4 cups (960 ml) filtered water
1 cup (130 g) raw pumpkin seeds
2 tablespoons agave nectar
¼ to ½ teaspoon vanilla extract or pulp from ½ vanilla bean, optional

1. Pour 2 cups (480 ml) of the water and the pumpkin seeds into a blender and blend until smooth. Add the agave nectar and vanilla, if using, and, with the blender running, slowly add the remaining 2 cups (480 ml) water. Blend until smooth.

2. Refrigerate until chilled. Pumpkin seed milk can be stored for up to 4 days in an airtight container in the refrigerator.

PER SERVING (1 CUP/240 ML) Calories: 210; total fat: 16 g; saturated fat: 3 g; cholesterol: 0 mg/dl; sodium: 0 mg; total carbohydrate: 12 g; dietary fiber: 2 g; sugar: 8 g; protein: 10 g; vitamin A: 0 mcg; vitamin C: 1.2 mg; calcium: 20 mg; iron: 2.7 mg
Rich in iron, phosphorus, magnesium, zinc, copper, and manganese

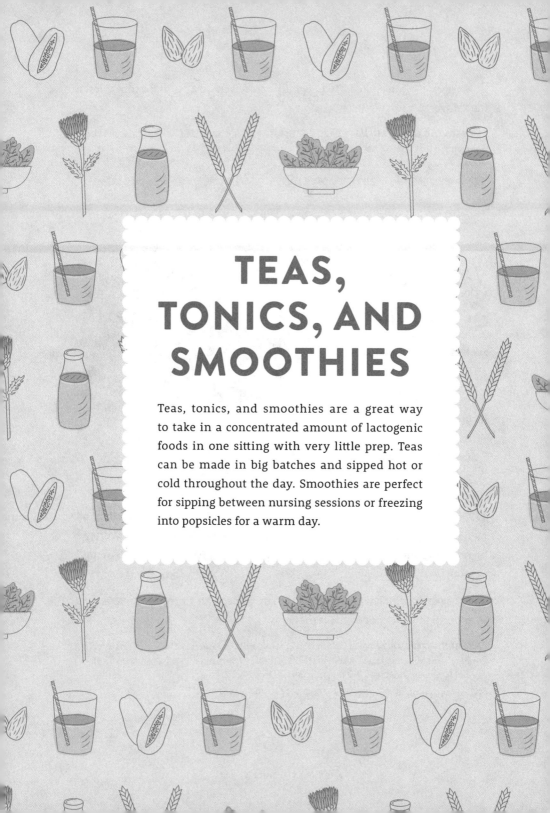

TEAS, TONICS, AND SMOOTHIES

Teas, tonics, and smoothies are a great way to take in a concentrated amount of lactogenic foods in one sitting with very little prep. Teas can be made in big batches and sipped hot or cold throughout the day. Smoothies are perfect for sipping between nursing sessions or freezing into popsicles for a warm day.

Golden Milk

MAKES 2 CUPS (480 ML)

MILK MAKERS: oats, barley

SUPERFOOD: turmeric

2 cups (480 ml) milk of choice
(preferably oat milk or barley milk)

1 teaspoon ground turmeric

2 to 3 teaspoons maple syrup
or agave nectar

2 teaspoons ginger juice (optional)

Whisk together all ingredients, including the ginger juice, if using, in a small saucepan. Cook over medium heat until warm.

PER SERVING (1 CUP/240 ML) Calories: 220; total fat: 2.5 g; saturated fat: 0 g; cholesterol: 0 mg/dl; sodium: 10 mg; total carbohydrate: 43 g; dietary fiber: 4 g; sugar: 18 g; protein: 7 g; vitamin A: 0 mcg; vitamin C: 0 mg; calcium: 60 mg; iron: 2.7 mg

Rich in iron, thiamin, riboflavin, phosphorus, magnesium, zinc, copper, and manganese

Fenugreek Tea

MAKES 1 CUP (240 ML)

MILK MAKER: fenugreek seeds

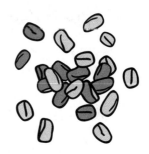

1 teaspoon whole fenugreek seeds

1 cup (240 ml) boiling water

1 to 2 teaspoons agave nectar

Steep the fenugreek seeds in boiling water for 10 minutes. Strain out the fenugreek and stir in the agave nectar to taste. Enjoy 3 to 4 times a day.

PER SERVING (1 CUP/240 ML) Calories: 45; total fat: 0 g; saturated fat: 0 g; cholesterol: 0 mg/dl; sodium: 0 mg; total carbohydrate: 11 g; dietary fiber: <1 g; sugar: 9 g; protein: 1 g; vitamin A: 0 mcg; vitamin C: 0 mg; calcium: 20 mg; iron: 1.5 mg

Milk Thistle Tea

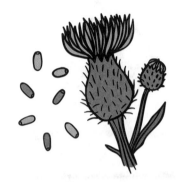

MAKES 1 CUP (240 ML)
MILK MAKER: milk thistle

1 teaspoon crushed milk thistle seeds
1 cup (240 ml) boiling water
1 to 2 teaspoons agave nectar

Steep the milk thistle seeds in the boiling water for 10 minutes. Strain out the milk thistle seeds and stir in the agave nectar to taste. Enjoy 2 to 3 times a day.

PER SERVING (1 CUP/240 ML) Calories: 45; total fat: 0 g; saturated fat: 0 g; cholesterol: 0 mg/dl; sodium: 10 mg; total carbohydrate: 12 g; dietary fiber: 1 g; sugar: 10 g; protein: 0 g; vitamin A: 0 mcg; vitamin C: 0 mg, calcium: 0 mg; iron: 0 mg

Barley Water

MAKES 3 CUPS (720 ML)
MILK MAKERS: barley, fennel seeds, fenugreek seeds

4 cups (960 ml) water
½ cup (100 g) pearled barley
2 to 3 teaspoons fennel seeds or 1 to 2 teaspoons fenugreek seeds, optional

Pour the water into a saucepan. Add the barley and seeds, if using, and simmer over medium heat for 10 minutes. Strain out the herbs (they usually float to the top). Simmer the barley for another 10 minutes. Strain out the barley and drink warm or cold.

VARIATION: If you have more time, use 1 cup (200 g) whole or pearled barley and simmer with 3 quarts (2.8 L) water for 2 hours, covered, over low heat. About half of the liquid should cook off. If the barley water becomes too thick to drink comfortably, add more water. Strain out the barley and drink warm or cold.

PER SERVING (1 CUP/240 ML) Calories: 10; total fat: 0 g; saturated fat: 0 g; cholesterol: 0 mg/dl; sodium: 0 mg; total carbohydrate: 3 g; dietary fiber: <1 g; sugar: 0 g; protein: 0 g; vitamin A: 0 mcg; vitamin C: 0 mg: calcium: 20 mg; iron: 0 mg

Barley Water Lemonade

MAKES 3 CUPS (720 ML)
MILK MAKER: barley

3 cups (720 ml) barley water (page 146)
Juice of 2 lemons (⅓ to ½ cup/80 to 120 ml)
¼ cup (60 ml) agave nectar

Stir the barley water, lemon juice, and agave nectar until the sweetener has completely dissolved. Pour into bottles and refrigerate until chilled.

PER SERVING (1 CUP/240 ML) Calories: 100; total fat: 0 g; saturated fat: 0 g; cholesterol: 0 mg/dl; sodium: 0 mg; total carbohydrate: 26 g; dietary fiber: 2 g; sugar: 21 g; protein: 0 g; vitamin A: 0 mcg; vitamin C: 12 mg; calcium: 20 mg; iron: 0 mg

Strawberry and Oats Smoothie

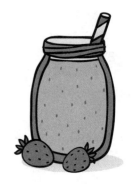

MAKES 1 SERVING

MILK MAKER: oats

SUPERFOODS: flaxseed, hemp, or chia oil

½ cup (120 ml) milk of choice

¼ cup (40 g) rolled oats

½ banana, broken into chunks

10 frozen strawberries

1 to 2 teaspoons agave nectar

2 teaspoons flaxseed, hemp, or chia oil

In a high-speed blender, blend all ingredients until smooth. Pour into a tall glass and serve immediately.

PER SERVING (2 CUPS/480 ML) Calories: 340; total fat: 15 g; saturated fat: 1.5 g; cholesterol: 0 mg/dl; sodium: 0 mg; total carbohydrate: 49 g; dietary fiber: 7 g; sugar: 23 g; protein: 7 g; vitamin A: 27.6 mcg; vitamin C: 48 mg; calcium: 20 mg; iron: 3 mg
Rich in vitamin C, iron, vitamin E, thiamin, riboflavin; vitamin B6, folate, phosphorus, magnesium, zinc, and manganese

Moringa-Berry Smoothie

MAKES 1 SERVING

MILK MAKER: moringa

SUPERFOODS: pumpkin seeds; flaxseed, hemp, or chia oil

1 cup (240 ml) mango nectar or juice

1 cup (140 g) frozen blueberries

1 cup (150 g) frozen strawberries

1 tablespoon pumpkin seed protein powder

1 teaspoon flaxseed, hemp, or chia oil

1 teaspoon moringa powder

1 tablespoon water or milk of choice (as needed)

Pour all the ingredients into a high-speed blender and blend until smooth. The smoothie may be very thick. To thin, add no more than 1 tablespoon water or milk.

PER SERVING (2 CUPS/480 ML) Calories: 350; total fat: 7 g; saturated fat: 0.5 g; cholesterol: 0 mg/dl; sodium: 60 mg; total carbohydrate: 68 g; dietary fiber: 10 g; sugar: 51 g; protein: 10 g; vitamin A: 1,932 mcg; vitamin C: 102 mg; calcium: 200 mg; iron: 6 mg

Rich in vitamin A, vitamin C, calcium, iron, vitamin E, vitamin K, folate, and manganese

Papaya Power Smoothie

MAKES 1 SERVING
MILK MAKERS: barley, papaya
SUPERFOOD: pumpkin seeds

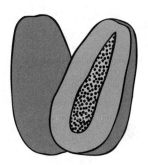

1 cup (240 ml) barley water (page 146)
¾ cup (105 g) frozen mango
¾ cup (130 g) frozen papaya
½ cup (75 g) frozen strawberries
¼ cup (65 g) raw pumpkin seeds
1 tablespoon agave nectar

Blend all the ingredients in a high-speed blender until smooth.

PER SERVING (2 CUPS/480 ML) Calories: 390; total fat: 16 g; saturated fat: 3 g; cholesterol: 0 mg/dl; sodium: 15 mg; total carbohydrate: 59 g; dietary fiber: 9 g; sugar: 43 g; protein: 11 g; vitamin A: 483 mcg; vitamin C: 102 mg, calcium: 80 mg; iron: 3.6 mg

Rich in vitamin A, vitamin C, iron, thiamin, niacin, folate, phosphorus, magnesium, zinc, copper, and manganese

BREAKFAST

As a dietitian, I see way too many people push breakfast aside each day. There isn't a reason I have not heard: "I'm too busy in the morning," "I feel sick when I eat in the morning," and "I'm just not hungry" are just the tip of the iceberg. However, as the adage goes, breakfast is the most important meal of the day. By the time breakfast rolls around, many have gone eight to twelve hours since their last meal. If you skip breakfast daily, that means you are going twelve to sixteen hours without eating each day! Just as your growing infant needs a healthy source of nutrients throughout the day to grow and thrive, you need a healthy source of nutrients throughout the day to ensure you have the calories to make enough milk for your infant and to nourish your body with the vitamins and minerals necessary for optimal health.

Granola

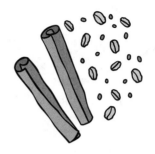

MAKES 3 CUPS (300 G)
MILK MAKER: oats
SUPERFOODS: hemp seeds, pumpkin seeds

3 cups (240 g) rolled oats

½ cup (80 g) organic raw, shelled hemp seeds

½ cup (65 g) pumpkin seeds

3 tablespoons light brown sugar

½ teaspoon ground cinnamon

⅛ teaspoon salt

⅓ cup (80 ml) agave nectar

¼ cup (60 ml) canola oil

1 teaspoon vanilla extract

1. Preheat the oven to 300°F (150°C) and line a baking sheet with parchment paper.

2. Combine the oats, hemp seeds, pumpkin seeds, brown sugar, cinnamon, and salt in a large bowl.

3. Whisk together the agave, canola oil, and vanilla extract in a separate small bowl.

4. Pour the agave mixture over the oat mixture and stir until the oats are completely coated. Spread the granola in a thin, even layer on the prepared baking sheet. Bake for 15 minutes, stir, and continue baking for 5 to 10 minutes more, until the granola is a light golden-brown color.

5. Remove the pan from the oven and allow to cool completely to room temperature. Once cooled, the granola will harden a bit. Break up any large chunks and store in an airtight container for up to 2 weeks.

PER SERVING (½ CUP/50 G) Calories: 100; total fat: 4.5 g; saturated fat: 0.5 g; cholesterol: 0 mg/dl; sodium: 10 mg; total carbohydrate: 12 g; dietary fiber: 2 g; sugar: 4 g; protein: 4 g; vitamin A: 0 mcg; vitamin C: 0 mg; calcium: 0 g; iron: 1 mg
Rich in phosphorus, magnesium, and manganese

Quick Coconut Milk Yogurt

MAKES 2 CUPS (250 G)
SUPERFOOD: probiotics

2 cups (200 g) fresh or frozen coconut meat
½ cup (120 ml) water or coconut water
2 teaspoons fresh lemon juice
1 probiotic capsule
½ teaspoon calcium carbonate powder
2 tablespoons sugar or agave nectar

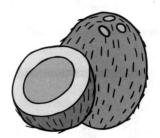

1. Blend all ingredients in a high-speed blender until smooth. Initially the yogurt will be a bit grainy; you will know it's perfect when it is completely smooth.

2. Transfer the yogurt to an airtight container, preferably glass, and refrigerate overnight or for at least 2 to 3 hours. The coconut yogurt will remain fresh in the refrigerator for 3 days.

PER SERVING (½ CUP/65 G) Calories: 170; total fat: 13 g; saturated fat: 12 g; cholesterol: 0 mg/dl; sodium: 40 mg; total carbohydrate: 14 g; dietary fiber: 4 g; sugar: 10 g; protein: 2 g; vitamin A: 0 mcg; vitamin C: 2.4 mg; calcium: 150 mg; iron: 1 mg
Rich in calcium, copper, and manganese

Sweet Potato Muffins

MAKES 12 MUFFINS
MILK MAKER: oats
SUPERFOODS: chia seeds, sweet potatoes, nuts

¼ cup (60 ml) water
1 tablespoon ground chia seeds
2 cups (210 g) oat flour (see page 135)
½ cup (100 g) sugar
1 tablespoon baking powder
2 teaspoons pumpkin pie spice
1 cup (200 g) mashed cooked sweet potato
1 cup (240 ml) milk of choice
¼ cup (65 g) nut butter of choice
1 tablespoon canola oil
1 teaspoon vanilla extract

1. Preheat the oven to 350°F (180°C) and line a 12-cup muffin pan with silicone or paper baking cups.

2. Whisk together the water and chia seeds in a small bowl; set aside.

3. Combine the oat flour, sugar, baking powder, and pumpkin pie spice in a large bowl. In a separate large bowl, stir together the sweet potato, milk, nut butter, canola oil, vanilla, and the chia seed mixture until combined.

4. Add the wet ingredients to the dry ingredients and stir until a cohesive dough forms. Divide the batter evenly among the prepared muffin cups and bake for 25 to 30 minutes, until a toothpick comes out clean.

PER MUFFIN Calories: 190; total fat: 7 g; saturated fat: 0.5 g; cholesterol: 0 mg/dl; sodium: 20 mg; total carbohydrate: 29 g; dietary fiber: 3 g; sugar: 10 g; protein: 6 g; vitamin A: 483 mcg; vitamin C: 1.2 mg; calcium: 100 mg; iron: 1.8 mg
Rich in vitamin A, calcium, iron, phosphorus, and manganese

Moringa Muffins

MAKES 12 MUFFINS
MILK MAKER: moringa
SUPERFOOD: chia seeds

¼ cup (60 ml) water
1 tablespoon ground chia seeds
½ cup (115 g) Earth Balance margarine, softened
½ cup (100 g) sugar
1 teaspoon vanilla extract
1½ cups (190 g) all-purpose flour
1 tablespoon baking powder
⅛ teaspoon fine salt
½ cup (120 ml) milk of choice
1 tablespoon white vinegar
3 teaspoons crushed dried moringa leaves or 2 teaspoons moringa powder

1. Preheat oven to 350°F (180°C). Line a 12-cup muffin pan with silicone or paper baking cups.

2. Whisk together the water and chia seeds in a small bowl; set aside.

3. Using an electric mixer, cream the softened margarine and sugar until light and fluffy. Beat in the chia seed mixture and vanilla extract. Stir in the flour, baking powder, and salt. Stir in the milk and vinegar until the batter is smooth. Then add the moringa and mix until combined. Fill the muffin cups about three-quarters full and bake for 18 to 20 minutes, until a toothpick inserted comes out clean.

PER MUFFIN Calories: 170; total fat: 8 g; saturated fat: 2 g; cholesterol: 0 mg/dl; sodium: 95 mg; total carbohydrate: 22 g; dietary fiber: <1 g; sugar: 9 g; protein: 2 g; vitamin A: 138 mcg; vitamin C: 0 mg; calcium: 80 mg; iron: 0.7 mg
Rich in phosphorus

Blueberry Avocado Muffins

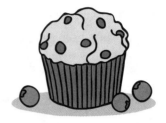

MAKES 12 MUFFINS
MILK MAKERS: whole wheat flour, oats
SUPERFOOD: avocado

MUFFINS

1 ripe avocado, peeled and pitted

½ cup (100 g) sugar

1 teaspoon vanilla extract

1 tablespoon white vinegar

1 cup (225 g) plain yogurt of choice

1 tablespoon baking powder

½ teaspoon baking soda

½ teaspoon salt

2 cups (240 g) whole wheat pastry flour

¾ cups (115 g) fresh or dried sweetened blueberries

STREUSEL TOPPING, OPTIONAL

¼ cup (20 g) rolled oats

¼ cup (50 g) sugar

2 tablespoons all-purpose flour

2 tablespoons Earth Balance margarine, melted

1. Preheat the oven to 375°F (190°C) and line a 12-cup muffin pan with silicone or paper baking cups.

2. Cream the avocado, sugar, and vanilla with an electric mixer until light and fluffy. Add the yogurt, baking powder, baking soda, and salt and mix to combine. Add the flour 1 cup at a time until the batter is just combined; then fold in the blueberries.

3. Divide the batter evenly among the prepared muffin cups.

4. To make the Streusel Topping, if using, stir together the oats, sugar, flour, and margarine and sprinkle evenly over each muffin.

RECIPE CONTINUES →

5. Bake for 20 to 25 minutes, until a toothpick comes out clean.

PER MUFFIN Calories: 190; total fat: 5 g; saturated fat: 1 g; cholesterol: <5 mg/dl; sodium: 180 mg; total carbohydrate: 34 g; dietary fiber: 4 g; sugar: 14 g; protein: 3 g; vitamin A: 0 mcg; vitamin C: 2.4 mg; calcium: 80 mg; iron: 0.7 mg
Rich in phosphorus

Hemp Seed Oatmeal

MAKES 2 SERVINGS
MILK MAKER: oats
SUPERFOOD: hemp seeds

2 cups (480 ml) water
1 cup (80 g) rolled oats
3 tablespoons brown sugar
3 tablespoons organic raw, shelled hemp seeds

1. In a small saucepan, bring the water to a boil. Add the oats, reduce the heat to low, and simmer uncovered for 10 minutes, or until the majority of the water has been absorbed and the oats are tender.

2. Turn off the heat and stir in the brown sugar and hemp seeds. Serve warm.

PER SERVING (1 CUP/235 G) Calories: 290; total fat: 9 g; saturated fat: 1.5 g; cholesterol: 0 mg/dl; sodium: 15 mg; total carbohydrate: 42 g; dietary fiber: 5 g; sugar: 14 g; protein: 10 g; vitamin A: 0 mcg; vitamin C: 0 mg; calcium: 20 mg; iron: 3.6 mg
Rich in iron, thiamin, phosphorus, magnesium, zinc, and manganese

All-Oats Waffles

MAKES 6 TO 8 WAFFLES
MILK MAKERS: oats, barley malt
SUPERFOOD: chia seeds

⅓ cup (80 ml) water

1 tablespoon ground chia seeds

1½ cups (160 g) oat flour (see page 135)

3 teaspoons baking powder

½ teaspoon salt

¼ teaspoon pumpkin pie spice

¾ cup (180 ml) milk of choice (preferably oat milk)

⅓ cup (80 ml) canola oil

2 tablespoons maple syrup (or 1 tablespoon maple syrup and 1 tablespoon barley malt)

1 tablespoon white vinegar

1 teaspoon vanilla extract

Nonstick cooking spray

1. Whisk together the water and chia seeds in a small bowl; set aside.

2. In a large bowl, whisk together the oat flour, baking powder, salt, and pumpkin pie spice. In a separate small bowl, whisk together the milk, canola oil, maple syrup, vinegar, vanilla, and the chia seed mixture.

3. Pour the wet ingredients into the dry ingredients. Stir until just combined. Let the batter rest uncovered for 5 to 10 minutes. While the batter is setting, preheat your waffle iron.

RECIPE CONTINUES →

4. Spray the waffle iron with nonstick cooking spray and ladle out ¼ cup (60 ml) of the batter at a time into the waffle molds. Cook until steam stops escaping from the iron, 3 to 5 minutes. Once the waffles are brown and crispy, transfer them to a cooling rack.

5. Repeat with the remaining batter.

PER WAFFLE (6 WAFFLES PER RECIPE; MADE WITH OAT MILK) Calories: 280; total fat: 15 g; saturated fat: 1.5 g; cholesterol: 0 mg/dl; sodium: 200 mg; total carbohydrate: 30 g; dietary fiber: 4 g; sugar: 6 g; protein: 6 g; vitamin A: 0 mcg; vitamin C: 0 mg; calcium: 150 mg; iron: 1.8 mg
Rich in vitamin E, vitamin K, phosphorus, and manganese

PER WAFFLE (8 WAFFLES PER RECIPE; MADE WITH OAT MILK) Calories: 210; total fat: 11 g; saturated fat: 1 g; 11 g; cholesterol: 0 mg/dl; sodium: 150 mg; total carbohydrate: 23 g; dietary fiber: 3 g; sugar: 4 g; protein: 5 g; vitamin A: 0 mcg; vitamin C: 0 mg; calcium: 100 mg; iron: 1.4 mg
Rich in calcium, iron, phosphorus, and manganese

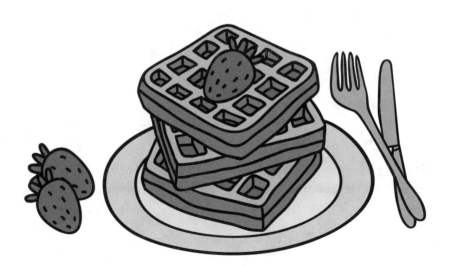

Power Pancakes

MAKES 24 SMALL PANCAKES
MILK MAKERS: oats, whole wheat, brewer's yeast
SUPERFOOD: chia seeds

½ cup (120 ml) water
2 tablespoons ground chia seeds
1 cup (105 g) oat flour (see page 135)
1 cup (120 g) whole wheat pastry flour
¼ cup (60 g) brewer's yeast
3 tablespoons baking powder
1 teaspoon baking soda
½ teaspoon ground cinnamon

½ teaspoon salt
¼ teaspoon ground nutmeg
2 cups (480 ml) milk of choice
¼ cup (60 ml) canola oil
3 tablespoons agave nectar
1 teaspoon vanilla extract
Nonstick cooking spray
Maple butter or pure maple syrup

1. Preheat an electric griddle to 375°F (190°C).

2. Whisk together the water and chia seeds in a small bowl; set aside.

3. Stir together the oat flour, whole wheat pastry flour, brewer's yeast, baking powder, baking soda, cinnamon, salt, and nutmeg in a large bowl. Whisk in the milk, oil, agave nectar, and vanilla until smooth and completely incorporated.

4. Lightly spray your hot griddle with nonstick cooking spray.

5. Use a ¼-cup (60 ml) measuring cup to scoop the pancake batter onto the griddle. Cook for 1 to 2 minutes on each side, until golden brown and cooked through. Serve warm with maple butter or maple syrup.

PER PANCAKE Calories: 90; total fat: 4 g; saturated fat: 0 g; cholesterol: 0 mg/dl; sodium: 105 mg; total carbohydrate: 12 g; dietary fiber: 2 g; sugar: 3 g; protein: 3 g; vitamin A: 0 mcg; vitamin C: 0 mg; calcium: 80 mg; iron: 0.7 mg
Rich in riboflavin and phosphorus

Oatmeal Pancakes

MAKES 12 PANCAKES

MILK MAKER: oats

SUPERFOODS: chia seeds, hemp seeds

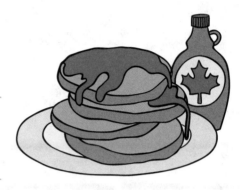

¼ cup (60 ml) water

1 tablespoon ground chia seeds

1¾ cups (185 g) oat flour (see page 135)

1 tablespoon plus 1 teaspoon baking powder

1 teaspoon sugar

¼ teaspoon salt

1 cup (240 ml) milk of choice

1½ tablespoons canola oil

1 tablespoon white vinegar

½ teaspoon vanilla extract

Nonstick cooking spray

Maple butter or pure maple syrup

1. Preheat an electric griddle to 375°F (190°C).

2. Whisk together the water and chia seeds in a small bowl; set aside.

3. Stir together the oat flour, baking powder, sugar, and salt in a large bowl. Add the milk, oil, vinegar, and vanilla. Whisk together until smooth.

4. Lightly spray your hot griddle with nonstick cooking spray.

5. Use a ¼-cup (60 ml) measuring cup to scoop the pancake batter onto the griddle. Cook for 1 to 2 minutes on each side, until golden brown and cooked through. Serve warm with maple butter or maple syrup.

PER PANCAKE Calories: 100; total fat: 4 g; saturated fat: 0 g; cholesterol: 0 mg/dl; sodium: 50 mg; total carbohydrate: 13 g; dietary fiber: 2 g; sugar: <1 g; protein: 4 g; vitamin A: 0 mcg; vitamin C: 0 mg; calcium: 80 mg; iron: 1.1 mg

Oatmeal Scones

MAKES 8 SCONES
MILK MAKER: oats

1⅔ cups (210 g) all-purpose flour
⅓ cup (75 g) packed light brown sugar
1 tablespoon baking powder
¾ teaspoon baking soda
¾ teaspoon pumpkin pie spice
½ teaspoon salt
1 ⅓ cups (110 g) rolled oats
¾ cup (170 g) cold Earth Balance margarine, cut into tablespoon pieces
⅔ cup (160 ml) milk of choice

1. Preheat the oven to 425°F (220°C) and line a baking sheet with parchment paper.

2. Pulse the flour, brown sugar, baking powder, baking soda, pumpkin pie spice, and salt in a food processor to combine. Add the oats and blend for 30 seconds. Add the margarine and pulse until the mixture resembles a coarse cornmeal; a few small lumps are OK.

3. Transfer to a large bowl. Add the milk and incorporate with a fork until a soft dough forms. Transfer the dough to the prepared baking sheet and form into a circle about ½ inch (13 mm) thick. Cut the circle into eight triangles.

4. Bake until the scones are golden brown and fluffy, 14 to 16 minutes. Remove from the oven and separate the scones, placing them about ½ inch (13 mm) apart. Bake for another 3 to 4 minutes, until golden brown.

PER SCONE Calories: 310; total fat: 17 g; saturated fat: 5 g; cholesterol: 0 mg/dl; sodium: 450 mg; total carbohydrate: 36 g; dietary fiber: 2 g; sugar: 10 g; protein: 4 g; vitamin A: 0 mcg; vitamin C: 0 mg; calcium: 100 mg; iron: 1.8 mg
Rich in calcium, iron, vitamin E, thiamin, folate, phosphorus, selenium, and manganese

Lemon Oat Scones

MAKES 8 SCONES
MILK MAKER: oats
SUPERFOODS: flaxseed, chia seeds

SCONES
¼ cup (60 ml) water
1 tablespoon ground flaxseed or ground chia seeds
2 cups (210 g) oat flour (see page 135)
1½ teaspoons cornstarch
½ teaspoon baking powder
½ teaspoon baking soda
¼ teaspoon salt
¼ cup (50 g) chia seeds
¼ cup (60 ml) agave nectar
¼ cup (60 g) Earth Balance margarine
1 tablespoon fresh lemon juice
½ teaspoon vanilla extract

LEMON GLAZE
¼ cup (30 g) confectioners' sugar
1 teaspoon fresh lemon juice

1. Preheat the oven to 350°F (180°C) and line a baking sheet with parchment paper.

2. Whisk together the water and flaxseed and set aside.

3. Combine the oat flour, cornstarch, baking powder, baking soda, and salt in a food processor and pulse ten times. Add the chia seeds and pulse an additional ten times.

4. Add the agave nectar, margarine, lemon juice, and vanilla to the food processor and process until a soft dough forms.

5. Transfer the dough to the prepared baking sheet and form into a circle about 1 inch (2.5 cm) thick. Cut into eight triangles.

6. Bake for 10 minutes. Remove from the oven and, using a sharp knife, separate the pieces. Bake for an additional 5 minutes. Cool on a wire rack while you prepare the glaze.

7. To make the Lemon Glaze, whisk the ingredients together and spoon over the scones once they have cooled slightly.

PER SCONE Calories: 250; total fat: 10 g; saturated fat: 2 g; cholesterol: 0 mg/dl; sodium: 200 mg; total carbohydrate: 35 g; dietary fiber: 6 g; sugar: 11 g; protein: 7 g; vitamin A: 0 mcg; vitamin C: 1.2 mg; calcium: 80 mg; iron: 1.8 mg
Rich in iron

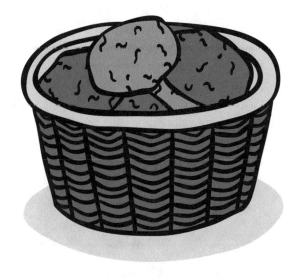

BREADS AND ROLLS

Oats and oatmeal tend to get a lot of credit for their milk-making abilities, but it's the beta-glucan in oats that helps raise serum prolactin levels and increases milk supply. One hundred percent whole-grain wheat, oats, and barley are all rich sources of beta-glucan, so having a peanut butter and jelly sandwich on whole wheat bread can go just as far as eating a bowl of oatmeal every morning. In this section I combine several varieties of beta-glucan-rich foods into homemade breads that pack a mighty prolactin punch.

Agave Graham Oatmeal Bread

MAKES 1 LOAF
MILK MAKERS: oats, barley, graham flour
SUPERFOOD: hemp seeds

2 cups (275 g) bread flour
1¼ cups (300 ml) milk of choice
1 cup (120 g) graham flour
1 cup (80 g) rolled oats
3 tablespoons agave nectar
2 tablespoons extra virgin olive oil
2 teaspoons bread machine yeast
1 teaspoon salt
3 tablespoons organic raw, shelled hemp seeds, optional

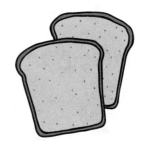

1. Place all the ingredients except the hemp seeds in the bowl of a bread machine. Program the machine for 1½ pounds (680 g) of bread on the dough cycle and press start. Fifteen minutes into the cycle, check the dough and scrape down the sides if any residual ingredients haven't been thoroughly mixed into the dough. Add the hemp seeds, if using, and continue to let the dough cycle run.

2. Once the dough cycle is complete (about 1½ hours), transfer the dough to an oiled 9 x 5-inch (23 x 13 cm) loaf pan. Cover the pan with a paper towel and set in a warm place to allow the dough to rise for 1 to 2 hours.

3. Preheat the oven to 350°F (180°C) and bake the bread for 30 to 35 minutes, until the bread makes a hollow sound when you tap it and the crust is deep brown. (Make sure to test for the hollow sound; it can look from the outside that it is cooked completely.)

RECIPE CONTINUES →

4. Remove the bread from the pan and allow to cool on a wire rack. Cool to room temperature and then slice as needed. The bread can be stored in the refrigerator for 3 to 5 days or in the freezer (slice it first) for up to 5 months.

PER SLICE (20 slices per recipe) Calories: 120; total fat: 3 g; saturated fat: 0 g; cholesterol: 0 mg/dl; sodium: 115 mg; total carbohydrate: 19 g; dietary fiber: 2 g; sugar: 3 g; protein: 4 g; vitamin A: 0 mcg; vitamin C: 0 mg; calcium: 0 mg; iron: 1.1 mg
Rich in thiamin and manganese

Barley Sandwich Bread

MAKES 1 LOAF
MILK MAKER: barley
SUPERFOOD: wheat germ

2 cups (275 g) bread flour

1¼ cups (300 ml) milk of choice

1 cup (125 g) all-purpose flour

½ cup (40 g) barley flakes

½ cup (60 g) barley flour

3 tablespoons olive oil

3 tablespoons toasted wheat germ

2 tablespoons agave nectar

1 tablespoon vital wheat gluten

2¼ teaspoons bread machine yeast

1 teaspoon sugar

¼ teaspoon baking soda

1 teaspoon salt

3 tablespoons organic raw, shelled hemp seeds, optional

1. Place all the ingredients except the hemp seeds in the bowl of a bread machine. Program the machine for 1½ pounds (680 g) of bread on the dough cycle and press start. Fifteen minutes into the cycle, check the dough and scrape down the sides if any residual ingredients haven't been thoroughly mixed into the dough. Add the hemp seeds, if using, and continue to let the dough cycle run.

2. Once the dough cycle is complete (about 1½ hours), transfer the dough to an oiled 9 x 5-inch (23 x 13 cm) loaf pan. Cover the pan with a paper towel and set in a warm place to allow the dough to rise for 30 to 60 minutes.

3. Preheat the oven to 350°F (180°C). Bake for 55 to 60 minutes, until the bottom sounds hollow when tapped. Check after 30 minutes and tent lightly if the top seems to be darkening too quickly.

4. Remove the bread from the pan and place on a wire rack to cool. Allow the loaf to sit for at least an hour before slicing.

PER SLICE (20 slices per recipe) Calories: 130; total fat: 3 g; saturated fat: 0 g; cholesterol: 0 mg/dl; sodium: 135 mg; total carbohydrate: 21 g; dietary fiber: 1 g; sugar: 2 g; protein: 4 g; vitamin A: 0 mcg; vitamin C: 0 mg; calcium: 0 mg; iron: 1.1 mg
Rich in thiamin and manganese

Pinto Bean Bread

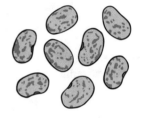

MAKES 1 LOAF
SUPERFOOD: pinto beans

2¾ cups (375 g) bread flour
1 cup (240 ml) milk of choice
1 cup (85 g) cooked pinto beans, mashed

1 tablespoon sugar
1 tablespoon canola oil
2½ teaspoons bread machine yeast
1 teaspoon salt

1. Place all the ingredients in the bowl of a bread machine. Program the machine for 1½ pounds (680 g) of bread on the dough cycle and press start. Fifteen minutes into the cycle, check the dough and scrape down the sides if any residual ingredients haven't been thoroughly mixed into the dough.

2. Once the dough cycle is complete (about 1½ hours), transfer the dough to an oiled 9 x 5-inch (23 x 13 cm) loaf pan. Cover the pan with a paper towel and set in a warm place to allow the dough to rise for 1 to 2 hours.

3. Preheat the oven to 350°F (180°C) and bake the bread for 35 to 40 minutes, until the bread makes a hollow sound when tapped and the crust is a deep brown.

PER SLICE (20 slices per recipe) Calories: 90; total fat: 1 g; saturated fat: 0 g; cholesterol: 0 mg/dl; sodium: 115 mg; total carbohydrate: 16 g; dietary fiber: 1 g; sugar: <1 g; protein: 3 g; vitamin A: 0 mcg; vitamin C: 0 mg; calcium: 0 mg; iron: 0.7 mg
Rich in thiamin

Beta Rolls

MAKES 20 TO 24 ROLLS

MILK MAKERS: oats, barley

2 cups (480 ml) warm water

1 cup (80 g) rolled oats

3 tablespoons Earth Balance margarine

2¼ teaspoons rapid-rising yeast or bread machine yeast

½ cup (120 ml) warm water

⅓ cup (75 g) packed brown sugar

1 teaspoon salt

2¼ cups (280 g) all-purpose flour

2 cups (240 g) barley flour

1. Bring the water to a boil in a medium saucepan. Add the oats and margarine and cook until the liquid is absorbed, about 10 minutes. Let cool.

2. Combine the cooked oats and the remaining ingredients in the bowl of a bread machine. Program the machine for 1½ pounds (680 g) of bread on the dough cycle and press start. Fifteen minutes into the cycle, check the dough and scrape down the sides if any residual ingredients haven't been thoroughly mixed into the dough.

3. Line two medium baking sheets with parchment paper. Once the dough cycle is complete (about 1½ hours), shape into 20 to 24 balls. The dough will be very sticky. Divide the balls between the two prepared baking sheets. Cover and let rise until doubled, about 45 minutes.

4. Preheat the oven to 350°F (180°C). Bake the rolls for 20 to 25 minutes, until golden brown.

PER ROLL (20 rolls per recipe) Calories: 150; total fat: 2.5 g; saturated fat: 0.5 g; cholesterol: 0 mg/dl; sodium: 135 mg; total carbohydrate: 28 g; dietary fiber: 2 g; sugar: 4 g; protein: 4 g; vitamin A: 0 mcg; vitamin C: 0 mg; calcium: 0 mg; iron: 1.4 mg
Rich in thiamin and selenium

Cornbread

MAKES 12 SERVINGS
MILK MAKERS: oats, barley
SUPERFOODS: hemp seeds, chia seeds

¼ cup (60 ml) water

1 tablespoon ground chia seeds

1 cup (130 g) cornmeal

1 cup (105 g) oat flour (see page 135) or barley flour

3 to 4 tablespoons sugar

1 teaspoon baking powder

½ teaspoon baking soda

½ teaspoon salt

1 cup (240 ml) milk of choice

½ cup (120 ml) canola oil

1 tablespoon white vinegar

2 tablespoons organic raw, shelled hemp seeds, optional

1. Preheat the oven to 375°F (190°C). Oil a 9-inch (23 cm) cast-iron skillet or baking dish.

2. Whisk together the water and chia seeds in a small bowl; set aside.

3. Whisk together the cornmeal, oat flour, sugar (more for sweeter cornbread), baking powder, baking soda, and salt in a large bowl. Add the milk, oil, and vinegar. Whisk until combined. Stir in the hemp seeds, if using.

4. Transfer the batter to the prepared skillet and bake for 20 to 25 minutes, until the bread begins to crack slightly and a toothpick comes out clean.

PER SLICE Calories: 190; total fat: 12 g; saturated fat: 1 g; cholesterol: 0 mg/dl; sodium: 150 mg; total carbohydrate: 19 g; dietary fiber: 2 g; sugar: 4 g; protein: 4 g; vitamin A: 0 mcg; vitamin C: 0 mg; calcium: 40 mg; iron: 1.4 mg
Rich in phosphorus and manganese

SIDE DISHES

Side dishes typically don't contain a large enough quantity of lactogenic foods or herbs to increase milk supply all on their own, but they're a great accompaniment to a meal that includes a lactogenic food as the main dish and as an addition to any other herbs or supplements you're taking.

Green Bean Coconut Curry

MAKES 6 SERVINGS
MILK MAKER: fenugreek seeds
SUPERFOOD: turmeric

1 tablespoon extra virgin olive oil

½ medium onion, sliced thin

1 garlic clove, minced

1 tablespoon curry powder

2 teaspoons fenugreek seeds

¼ teaspoon red pepper flakes, optional

¼ teaspoon ground turmeric

¼ teaspoon salt

1 pound (455 g) fresh or frozen and thawed
green beans

¾ cup (180 ml) coconut milk

½ to 1 tablespoon brown sugar

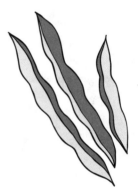

Heat the oil in a saucepan over medium-high heat. Cook the onion in the oil until it begins to brown, about 10 minutes. Add the garlic and cook an additional minute. Stir in the curry powder, fenugreek seeds, red pepper flakes, if using, turmeric, and salt; cook for another 3 minutes. Add the green beans and stir until evenly coated. Pour in the coconut milk and brown sugar and simmer for at least 5 minutes but up to 30 minutes.

PER SERVING Calories: 130; total fat: 10 g; saturated fat: 7 g; cholesterol: 0 mg/dl; sodium: 110 mg; total carbohydrate: 11 g; dietary fiber: 4 g; sugar: 5 g; protein: 3 g; vitamin A: 138 mcg; vitamin C: 12 mg; calcium: 40 mg; iron: 1.8 mg
Rich in vitamin A, iron, vitamin K, magnesium, and manganese

Baked Avocado Fries

MAKES 4 TO 6 SERVINGS
SUPERFOOD: avocado

2 ripe avocados, peeled and pitted
¼ cup (30 g) all-purpose flour
½ cup (120 ml) milk of choice
¼ cup (15 g) plain instant potato flakes
⅔ cup (80 g) plain bread crumbs
½ teaspoon garlic powder
¼ teaspoon salt
Nonstick cooking spray

1. Preheat the oven to 425°F (220°C). Line a baking sheet with parchment paper.

2. Cut the avocado into strips about ½ inch (13 mm) thick. Place in a shallow bowl and toss to coat with the flour. Whisk together the milk and potato flakes in a small shallow bowl. Stir together the bread crumbs, garlic powder, and salt in a separate small shallow bowl.

3. Dredge the flour-dusted avocado in the milk mixture and then in the bread-crumbs, pressing the avocado into the bread crumbs to coat each slice completely. Place the avocado slices in a single layer on the prepared baking sheet, spray with cooking spray, and bake for 15 minutes or until the fries are golden brown. Serve with a dip of your choice!

PER SERVING (6 SERVINGS PER RECIPE) Calories: 130; total fat: 8 g; saturated fat: 1 g; cholesterol: 0 mg/dl; sodium: 125 mg; total carbohydrate: 13 g; dietary fiber: 4 g; sugar: <1 g; protein: 3 g; vitamin A: 27.6 mcg; vitamin C: 6 mg; calcium: 20 mg; iron: <1 mg
Rich in vitamin K, thiamin, folate, and manganese

Ginger-Glazed Carrots

MAKES 4 SERVINGS
SUPERFOOD: carrots

8 carrots, peeled
3 tablespoons extra virgin olive oil
Pinch of salt, or to taste
2½ tablespoons agave nectar
¼ teaspoon ground ginger
⅛ teaspoon ground cloves

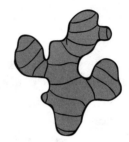

1. Preheat the oven to 350°F (180°C). Line a baking dish with parchment paper.

2. Place the whole carrots in the prepared baking dish and drizzle with the olive oil. Mix until the carrots are completely covered and evenly coated. Sprinkle lightly with the salt.

3. Bake the carrots for about 30 minutes, until just tender. Whisk together the agave nectar, ginger, and cloves. Remove the carrots from the oven and baste with the ginger mixture, bake for an additional 5 minutes.

PER SERVING Calories: 180; total fat: 11 g; saturated fat: 1.5 g; cholesterol: 0 mg/dl; sodium: 125 mg; total carbohydrate: 22 g; dietary fiber: 4 g; sugar: 15 g; protein: 1 g; vitamin A: 5,658 mcg; vitamin C: 6 mg; calcium: 40 mg; iron: <1 mg
Rich in vitamin A, vitamin K, and manganese

Spinach and Sweet Potato Curry with Caramelized Onions

MAKES 6 SERVINGS
SUPERFOODS: sweet potato, spinach, peanuts

1 tablespoon extra virgin olive oil

1 small sweet onion, sliced thin

⅔ cup (160 ml) vegetable broth

3 tablespoons red curry paste

2 medium sweet potatoes, peeled and cubed

One 13.5-ounce (400 ml) can regular coconut milk

4 cups (80 g) fresh baby spinach

½ cup (75 g) chopped peanuts

2 tablespoons chopped fresh cilantro

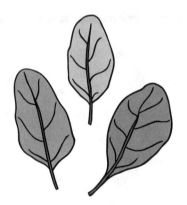

1. Warm the oil over medium-high heat in a medium stockpot. Add the onion and toss to coat with oil. Cook for 20 to 30 minutes, until the onion is a deep golden brown, stirring every 5 minutes and checking often so they don't burn (see Note). Deglaze the pan by pouring in the broth and stirring while scraping down the sides of the skillet. Add the curry paste and stir to combine. Add the sweet potatoes and coconut milk. Cook on medium heat for 15 minutes, or until the potatoes are tender.

2. Stir in the spinach and cook until wilted. Before serving, top with the peanuts and cilantro.

NOTE: The longer you're able to cook the onion, the richer the end product will be; however, if you're short on time, cook the onion for at least 15 minutes.

PER SERVING Calories: 280; total fat: 20 g; saturated fat: 11 g; cholesterol: 0 mg/dl; sodium: 390 mg; total carbohydrate: 21 g; dietary fiber: 4 g; sugar: 7 g; protein: 7 g; vitamin A: 3,450 mcg; vitamin C: 21 mg; calcium: 100 mg; iron: 3.6 mg

Rich in vitamin A, calcium, iron, vitamin K, vitamin B6, folate, magnesium, copper, and manganese

Fried Green Papaya with Smoky Cilantro Remoulade

MAKES 6 SERVINGS

MILK MAKER: green papaya

SMOKY CILANTRO REMOULADE

1 cup Just Mayo

3 tablespoons Dijon mustard

2 to 3 tablespoons chopped fresh cilantro

1 garlic clove, minced

1 tablespoon fresh lime juice

2 teaspoons capers with juice, chopped

1 teaspoon Cajun seasoning

1 teaspoon hot sauce

1 teaspoon smoked paprika

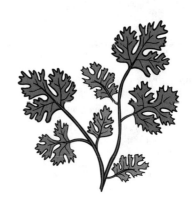

FRIED GREEN PAPAYA

1 large green papaya, sliced into ¼-inch (6 mm) thick medallions

1 cup (125 g) all-purpose flour

⅔ cup (160 ml) milk of choice

¼ cup (15 g) instant potato flakes

½ cup (60 g) cornmeal

½ cup (60 g) plain bread crumbs

1 tablespoon Cajun seasoning, optional

Canola oil for frying

RECIPE CONTINUES →

1. **To make the Smoky Cilantro Remoulade,** mix together all of the ingredients in a small bowl. Allow to chill in the refrigerator for 1 hour for the flavors to meld.

2. **To make the Fried Green Papaya,** bring a pot of water to a boil. Add the papaya to the water. Cover and cook over medium-high heat until just tender, 5 to 8 minutes. Remove the papaya from the pot and cool under cold water.

3. Place the flour in a shallow bowl. Whisk together the milk and potato flakes in another shallow bowl. Combine the cornmeal, bread crumbs, and Cajun seasoning in a third shallow bowl. You should have three bowls sitting next to each other—one with flour, one with the milk mixture, and one with the cornmeal mixture.

4. Dip the papaya in the flour until coated, then in the milk, and finally in the cornmeal, turning to coat.

5. Fill a heavy-bottomed pan such as a cast-iron skillet with ½ inch (13 mm) of canola oil. Warm over medium to medium-high heat. Fry the papaya in batches, 3 to 5 minutes per side, until golden brown and crispy. Drain on paper towels. Serve with the remoulade.

PER SERVING Calories: 550; total fat: 38 g; saturated fat: 3.5 g; cholesterol: 0 mg/dl; sodium: 3,100 mg; total carbohydrate: 47 g; dietary fiber: 3 g; sugar: 8 g; protein: 5 g; vitamin A: 276 mcg; vitamin C: 36 mg, calcium: 40 mg; iron: 2.7 mg
Rich in vitamin K, thiamin, phosphorus, selenium, and manganese

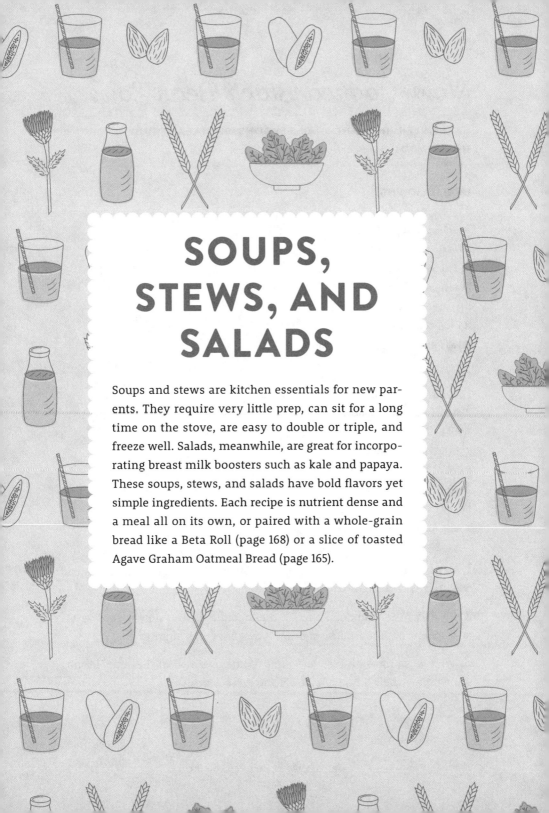

SOUPS, STEWS, AND SALADS

Soups and stews are kitchen essentials for new parents. They require very little prep, can sit for a long time on the stove, are easy to double or triple, and freeze well. Salads, meanwhile, are great for incorporating breast milk boosters such as kale and papaya. These soups, stews, and salads have bold flavors yet simple ingredients. Each recipe is nutrient dense and a meal all on its own, or paired with a whole-grain bread like a Beta Roll (page 168) or a slice of toasted Agave Graham Oatmeal Bread (page 165).

Slow-Cooked Black Bean Soup

MAKES 8 SERVINGS AND 7 TABLESPOONS (55 G) SEASONING
SUPERFOODS: beans, carrots

TACO SEASONING

3 tablespoons chili powder

2 tablespoons ground cumin

2 teaspoons paprika

1 teaspoon garlic powder

1 teaspoon onion powder

1 teaspoon salt

½ teaspoon black pepper

¼ teaspoon cayenne powder, optional

SOUP

1 pound (455 g) dried black beans, soaked overnight

2 medium carrots, peeled and diced

½ medium onion, diced

2 garlic cloves, minced

4 cups (960 ml) vegetable broth

3 cups (720 ml) water

1 cup (240 ml) medium salsa

½ teaspoon hickory liquid smoke

1. **To make the Taco Seasoning,** mix together all the ingredients in a small container with a lid for storing (see Note).

2. **To make the Soup,** combine all the ingredients in a slow cooker with 2 tablespoons of the Taco Seasoning and cook for 6 to 8 hours on low.

3. With an immersion blender, puree a little over half of the soup, leaving some beans whole. Ladle into bowls and serve warm.

NOTE: Use leftover seasoning in Lentil Tacos (page 200) or Chia-Flecked Empanadas (page 202).

TACO SEASONING: PER SERVING (1 TABLESPOON) Calories: 20; total fat: 1 g; saturated fat: 0 g; cholesterol: 0 mg/dl; sodium: 470 mg; total carbohydrate: 4 g; dietary fiber: 2 g; sugar: 0 g; protein: 1 g; vitamin A: 405 mcg; vitamin C: 0 mg; calcium: 26 mg; iron: 1.8 mg
Rich in iron and vitamin A

SOUP: PER SERVING Calories: 230; total fat: 1 g; saturated fat: 0 g; cholesterol: 0 mg/dl; sodium: 350 mg; total carbohydrate: 44 g; dietary fiber: 11 g; sugar: 4 g; protein: 14 g; vitamin A: 900 mcg; vitamin C: 5 mg; calcium: 104 mg; iron: 4.5 mg
Rich in iron, calcium, potassium, vitamin A, thiamin, vitamin B6, folate, phosphorus, magnesium, zinc, copper, and manganese

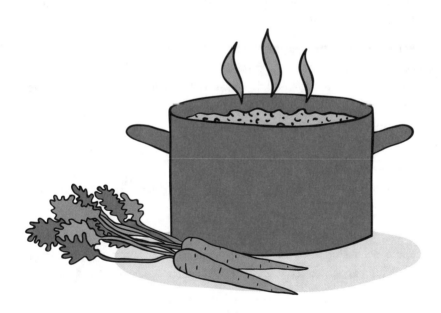

Roasted Carrot Soup

MAKES 4 SERVINGS
SUPERFOODS: carrots, turmeric

8 large carrots, peeled

4 tablespoons extra virgin olive oil

Pinch of salt

½ large sweet onion, chopped

2 large garlic cloves, chopped

2 teaspoons ground turmeric

6 cups (1.4 L) vegetable broth

1-inch (2.5 cm) piece fresh ginger, or 1 tablespoon ginger juice

1 thyme sprig, plus more for garnish

Freshly ground black pepper

1. Preheat the oven to 350°F (180°C).

2. Place the carrots in a baking dish and drizzle with 2 tablespoons of the olive oil. Mix until the carrots are completely coated. Sprinkle lightly with salt. Bake until tender, 25 to 30 minutes.

3. While the carrots are roasting, warm the remaining 2 tablespoons of oil in a medium stockpot over medium-high heat. Add the onion and cook until translucent, 3 to 5 minutes. Add the garlic and cook for an additional minute. Stir in the turmeric and coat the onion and garlic. Add the vegetable broth, ginger, and thyme. Bring the broth to a boil and simmer gently for 15 minutes.

4. Add the cooked carrots to the stockpot. Remove the ginger and thyme from the broth. Simmer for 5 to 10 minutes, until the carrots are soft enough to puree.

5. Use an immersion or a standard blender to puree the mixture until smooth. If the soup seems too thick, add more broth or water and reheat gently. Season with salt and pepper. To serve, garnish with chopped fresh thyme.

PER SERVING Calories: 230; total fat: 15 g; saturated fat: 2 g; cholesterol: 0 mg/dl; sodium: 350 mg; total carbohydrate: 24 g; dietary fiber: 6 g; sugar: 13 g; protein: 3 g; vitamin A: 7,200 mcg; vitamin C: 14 mg; calcium: 104 mg; iron: 1.8 mg
Rich in calcium, iron, potassium, vitamin A, vitamin C, vitamin K, vitamin B6, and manganese

Dashi Ramen Soup

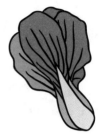

MAKES 2 SERVINGS
MILK MAKER: mushrooms
SUPERFOODS: miso, seaweed, bok choy

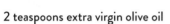

2 teaspoons extra virgin olive oil

3 ounces (85 g) shiitake mushrooms

2 heads baby bok choy, sliced thin

4 cups (960 ml) water

2-inch (5 cm) piece dried kombu

1 tablespoon sweet miso paste

12 ounces (340 g) fresh or dried ramen noodles

Warm the oil in a medium saucepan and sauté the mushrooms and bok choy until tender. Stir in the water, kombu, and miso paste and bring to a low boil. Add the ramen noodles and simmer uncovered for 3 to 4 minutes, until the noodles are al dente. Ladle the soup into bowls and serve warm.

PER SERVING Calories: 750; total fat: 9 g; saturated fat: 1 g; cholesterol: 0 mg/dl; sodium: 1,200 mg; total carbohydrate: 147 g; dietary fiber: 26 g; sugar: 6 g; protein: 31 g; vitamin A: 990 mcg; vitamin C: 36 mg; calcium: 195 mg; iron: 9 mg
Rich in calcium, vitamin A, vitamin C, pantothenic acid, and copper

Moroccan Spiced Chickpea Stew

MAKES 6 SERVINGS
SUPERFOODS: chickpeas, spinach

3 tablespoons extra virgin olive oil

½ medium onion, diced

6 garlic cloves, minced

1 teaspoon ground cumin

1 teaspoon paprika

½ teaspoon ground cinnamon

⅛ teaspoon cayenne pepper

4½ cups (740 g) cooked chickpeas

4 cups (960 ml) vegetable broth

One 14.5-ounce (410 g) can chopped tomatoes

1 teaspoon sugar

1 cup (155 g) frozen spinach

RECIPE CONTINUES →

Warm the oil in a large stockpot over medium heat. Add the onion and cook until translucent, about 5 minutes. Add the garlic and cook until fragrant, about 1 minute. Add the cumin, paprika, cinnamon, and cayenne pepper and stir for an additional minute. Stir in the chickpeas, broth, tomatoes, and sugar. Simmer, covered, for 30 minutes. Stir in the spinach and simmer for an additional 15 minutes.

PER SERVING Calories: 310; total fat: 10 g; saturated fat: 1.5 g; cholesterol: 0 mg/dl; sodium: 780 mg; total carbohydrate: 43 g; dietary fiber: 12 g; sugar: 10 g; protein: 13 g; vitamin A: 1,170 mcg; vitamin C: 14 mg; calcium: 130 mg; iron: 4.5 mg
Rich in calcium, iron, vitamin A, vitamin C, vitamin E, vitamin K, thiamin, vitamin B6, folate, phosphorus, magnesium, zinc, copper, and manganese

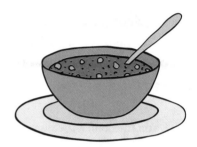

Vegetable and Barley Stew

MAKES 8 SERVINGS
MILK MAKERS: barley, fenugreek seeds
SUPERFOODS: carrots, chickpeas

2 quarts (2 L) vegetable broth

2 large carrots, chopped

2 celery stalks, chopped

One 14.5-ounce (410 g) can diced tomatoes with juice

One 15-ounce (425 g) can chickpeas, rinsed and drained

1 onion, chopped

1 cup (200 g) pearl barley

2 teaspoons fenugreek seeds

1 teaspoon curry powder

1 teaspoon garlic powder

1 teaspoon paprika

1 teaspoon sugar

1 teaspoon vegan Worcestershire sauce

¼ teaspoon ground black pepper

3 bay leaves

Combine all the ingredients in a large stockpot and bring to a boil. Cover and simmer over medium-low heat for 1½ hours. The soup will be very thick. You may adjust by adding more broth, if desired. Remove the bay leaves before serving.

NOTE: This recipe can also be made in a slow cooker. Combine all ingredients in a slow cooker, cover, and cook on low for 8 hours. Stir in plain warm barley water (page 146) or broth to thin out the soup, if you desire.

PER SERVING Calories: 230; total fat: 2 g; saturated fat: 0 g; cholesterol: 0 mg/dl; sodium: 1,230 mg; total carbohydrate: 50 g; dietary fiber: 11 g; sugar: 6 g; protein: 7 g; vitamin A: 1,350 mcg; vitamin C: 18 mg; calcium: 130 mg; iron: 6.3 mg
Rich in calcium, iron, vitamin A, vitamin C, vitamin B6, folate, magnesium, zinc, selenium, copper, and manganese

Spring Salad with Balsamic Vinaigrette and Spiced Pecans

MAKES 4 SERVINGS AND 1¾ CUPS (420 ML) VINAIGRETTE
SUPERFOODS: green leafy vegetables, carrots, flaxseed oil, pecans

SPICED PECANS
1 cup (240 ml) warm water
¼ cup (50 g) plus 2 tablespoons sugar

1 cup (100 g) pecan halves
1 tablespoon chili powder

BALSAMIC VINAIGRETTE
½ cup (120 ml) balsamic vinegar
½ cup (120 ml) extra virgin olive oil
½ cup (120 ml) flaxseed oil

3 tablespoons agave nectar
2 tablespoons Dijon mustard
2 garlic cloves, minced

RECIPE CONTINUES →

SPRING SALAD

One 11-ounce (312 g) can mandarin oranges in juice, drained

1 head romaine lettuce, sliced thin, or 6 ounces (170 g) fresh baby salad greens

1 pint (285 g) cherry or grape tomatoes

½ cup (55 g) shredded carrots

1. **To make the Spiced Pecans,** combine the water and ¼ cup (50 g) of the sugar in a bowl. Add the pecan halves and soak for 10 minutes. Preheat the oven to 350°F (180°C) and lightly grease a baking sheet.

2. Drain the pecans and discard the sugar water. Combine the remaining 2 tablespoons of sugar and chili powder. Toss with the pecans and place on the baking sheet. Bake for 10 to 15 minutes, until golden brown, stirring once. Remove from the oven and allow to cool in the pan.

3. **To make the Balsamic Vinaigrette,** whisk together all the ingredients, transfer to an airtight container, and store in the refrigerator until ready to use. The vinaigrette can be refrigerated for up to 7 days.

4. **To make the Spring Salad,** combine all the ingredients together in a large serving bowl. Toss with the Balsamic Vinaigrette and top with the Spiced Pecans.

SPICED PECANS: PER SERVING (¼ CUP/45 G) Calories: 250; total fat: 18 g; saturated fat: 1.5 g; cholesterol: 0 mg/dl; sodium: 85 mg; total carbohydrate: 23 g; dietary fiber: 3 g; sugar: 20 g; protein: 3 g; vitamin A: 180 mcg; vitamin C: 0 mg; calcium: 26 mg; iron 1.1 mg
Rich in vitamin A, thiamin, zinc, copper, and manganese

BALSAMIC VINAIGRETTE: PER SERVING (1 TABLESPOON)
Calories: 80; total fat: 7 g; saturated fat: 1 g; cholesterol: 0 mg/dl; sodium: 10 mg; total carbohydrate: 2 g; dietary fiber: 0 g; sugar: 2 g; protein: 0 g; vitamin A: 0 mcg; vitamin C: 0 mg; calcium: 0 mg; iron: 0 mg

Spicy Wilted Kale Salad

MAKES 4 SERVINGS
SUPERFOODS: kale, carrot, pecans

4 cups (65 g) thinly sliced kale
1 medium carrot, peeled and grated
½ cup (50 g) chopped pecans
½ cup (110 g) Just Mayo
¼ cup (40 g) golden raisins
2 tablespoons sugar
1 tablespoon raw apple cider vinegar
½ teaspoon dried oregano
½ teaspoon dried thyme
½ teaspoon ground allspice
½ teaspoon paprika
¼ teaspoon curry powder
¼ teaspoon salt
⅛ teaspoon cayenne pepper
⅛ teaspoon ground cinnamon
⅛ teaspoon ground cloves
⅛ teaspoon ground nutmeg

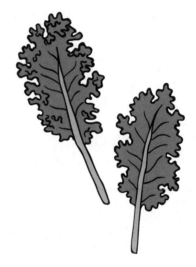

Combine all the ingredients in a large bowl and toss until the kale is evenly covered. Cover and chill for at least 1 hour before serving.

PER SERVING Calories: 370; total fat: 31 g; saturated fat: 3 g; cholesterol: 0 mg/dl; sodium: 340 mg; total carbohydrate: 26 g; dietary fiber: 5 g; sugar: 15 g; protein: 5 g; vitamin A: 2,790 mcg; vitamin C: 81 mg; calcium: 130 mg; iron: 1.8 mg
Rich in calcium, iron, vitamin A, vitamin K, thiamin, vitamin B6, folate, magnesium, copper, and manganese

Caesar Salad with Falafel Chickpeas

MAKES 4 SERVINGS AND 1 CUP (240 ML) DRESSING
SUPERFOODS: hemp oil, flaxseed oil, chickpeas, romaine lettuce

CAESAR DRESSING
½ cup (110 g) Just Mayo
Juice of 1 large lemon (about ¼ cup/60 ml)
3 tablespoons nutritional yeast
1½ tablespoons capers
1 tablespoon whole-grain mustard
1 teaspoon Dijon mustard
2 garlic cloves, chopped
¼ teaspoon vegan Worcestershire sauce
¼ teaspoon black pepper
¼ teaspoon salt
¼ cup (60 ml) hemp or flaxseed oil
1 tablespoon organic raw, shelled hemp seeds

SALAD
Two heads romaine lettuce, rinsed and roughly chopped
1 batch Falafel Roasted Chickpeas (page 195)

1. **To make the Caesar Dressing,** blend the mayo, lemon juice, nutritional yeast, capers, mustards, garlic, Worcestershire sauce, pepper, and salt in a blender or food processor until creamy and smooth. With the blender still running, slowly add the oil. Stir in the hemp seeds.

2. **To make the Salad,** place the lettuce in a large bowl and add the Caesar dressing 2 tablespoons at a time, incorporating with a spatula until every leaf is covered with dressing (but not drenched). Sprinkle with the roasted chickpeas and serve.

CAESAR DRESSING: PER SERVING (¼ CUP/60 ML) Calories: 360; total fat: 35 g; saturated fat: 3 g; cholesterol: 0 mg/dl; sodium: 880 mg; total carbohydrate: 8 g; dietary fiber: 2 g; sugar: 0 g; protein: 5 g; vitamin A: 0 mcg; vitamin C: 7 mg; calcium: 0 mg; iron: 0.7 mg
Rich in thiamin, riboflavin, niacin, vitamin B6, folate, vitamin B12, and zinc

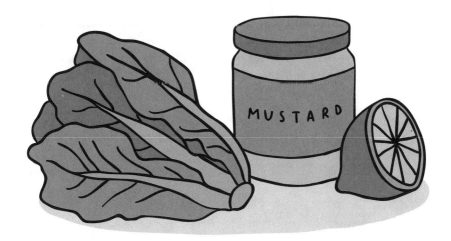

Green Papaya Salad Som Tum

MAKES 2 SMALL SALADS
MILK MAKER: papaya

5 cherry tomatoes

5 fresh green beans

2 chile peppers, such as Thai chiles, serrano chiles, or jalapeños

1 garlic clove, sliced thin

1-inch (2.5 cm) piece fresh ginger, grated, or 1 tablespoon ginger juice

2 cups (280 g) shredded green papaya

Juice of 1 lime

1½ tablespoons sugar

2 teaspoons Bragg liquid aminos

¼ cup (35 g) toasted peanuts

With the back of a large spoon, crush the tomatoes, green beans, chiles, garlic, and ginger in a large bowl. You can also use a large mortar and pestle. Add the shredded papaya, lime juice, sugar, and liquid aminos and toss to coat. Sprinkle with the peanuts. Serve cold.

PER SERVING Calories: 240; total fat: 10 g; saturated fat: 1.5 g; cholesterol: 0 mg/dl; sodium: 340 mg; total carbohydrate: 38 mg; dietary fiber: 6 g; sugar: 25 g; protein: 7 g; vitamin A: 630 mcg; vitamin C: 207 mg; calcium: 52 mg; iron: 1.4 mg
Rich in potassium, vitamin C, vitamin A, vitamin E, thiamin, niacin, vitamin B6, folate, magnesium, copper, and manganese

DIPS, BARS, AND SNACKS

The average breastfeeding mother will burn somewhere between 400 and 600 calories a day nursing her little one on demand. That is as much as an hour-long spin class or a two-hour hike! Your body is using a lot of energy to make milk for your little one, and many mothers feel hungry and thirsty immediately after nursing or will have spikes of extreme hunger during the day or in the middle of the night. Keeping healthy snacks on hand is the key to maintaining a healthy diet while your body tries to adjust and provide for your little one. You want to choose snacks that have a source of lean protein such as beans, nuts, or seeds; healthy fats such as avocado or almonds; and whole grains to give your body and brain the immediate energy it needs. Each of these snacks is equipped with just the right amount of protein, fat, and carbs you need to feel full and satisfied between nursing sessions while helping to build and maintain a healthy milk supply.

Classic Hummus

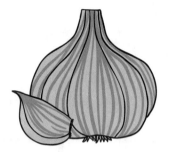

MAKES 3 CUPS (740 G)
SUPERFOODS: chickpeas, flaxseed oil, hemp oil

1 head garlic
1 teaspoon extra virgin olive oil
3 cups (495 g) cooked chickpeas
⅓ cup (80 ml) water
¼ cup (60 g) tahini
¼ cup (60 ml) flaxseed oil or hemp oil (or a combination of both)
Juice of ½ lemon (about 1½ tablespoons)
¾ teaspoon salt

1. Preheat the oven to 400°F (200°C).

2. Peel away the outer layers of the garlic bulb skin, leaving the skins of the individual cloves intact. Cut off ¼ inch (6 mm) from the top of cloves, exposing the individual cloves of garlic.

3. Place the garlic head in a baking pan and drizzle with the olive oil, using your fingers to make sure the garlic head is well coated. Cover with aluminum foil. Bake for 30 to 35 minutes, until the cloves feel soft when pressed.

4. Allow the garlic to cool enough so you can touch it without burning yourself. Use a paring knife to cut the skin slightly around each clove. Use your fingers to pull or squeeze the roasted garlic cloves out of their skins.

5. Combine the garlic and the remaining ingredients in a food processor and process until smooth and fluffy. Store in an airtight container in the refrigerator for up to 4 days.

PER SERVING (½ CUP/125 G) Calories: 290; total fat: 17 g; saturated fat: 2 g; cholesterol: 0 mg/dl; sodium: 300 mg; total carbohydrate: 26 g; dietary fiber: 7 g; sugar: 4 g; protein: 9 g; vitamin A: 0 mcg; vitamin C: 4 mg; calcium: 52 mg; iron: 2.7 mg
Rich in iron, vitamin E, thiamin, vitamin B6, folate, phosphorous, magnesium, zinc, selenium, copper, and manganese

New Mom Guacamole

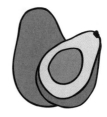

MAKES 1 CUP (300 G)
SUPERFOOD: avocado

2 ripe Hass avocados, halved and
pitted

Juice of ½ lime

1 tablespoon dried cilantro (or 3
tablespoons fresh)

½ teaspoon salt

¼ teaspoon garlic powder

Scoop the avocado flesh into a medium bowl and mash with the back of a large
spoon. Add the lime juice, cilantro, salt, and garlic powder. Stir to combine.

PER SERVING (¼ CUP/75 G) Calories: 120; total fat: 10 g; saturated fat: 1.5 g; cholesterol:
0 mg/dl; sodium: 300 mg; total carbohydrate: 7 g; dietary fiber: 5 g; sugar: 0 g; protein: 1 g;
vitamin A: 54 mcg; vitamin C: 7 mg; calcium: 0 mg; iron: 0.4 mg
Rich in vitamin E, vitamin K, vitamin B6, folate, pantothenic acid, and copper

Peanut Butter Barley Treats

MAKES 4 SERVINGS
MILK MAKERS: barley, barley malt
SUPERFOOD: peanuts

1½ tablespoons Earth Balance
margarine

2 tablespoons barley malt or agave
nectar

¼ cup (65 g) creamy peanut butter

1¼ cups (20 g) puffed barley cereal

1. In a small saucepan over medium heat, melt the margarine. Stir in the barley
malt. Add the peanut butter, stirring as it continues softening. Once everything
is fully melted, 3 to 5 minutes, remove the pan from the heat and stir in the
puffed barley cereal.

RECIPE CONTINUES →

2. Scoop dollops of the mixture into mini muffin cups and set the cups on a plate or tray. Place the plate with the cups in the refrigerator and chill until firm, about an hour. Enjoy!

PER SERVING Calories: 190; total fat: 12 g; saturated fat: 3 g; cholesterol: 0 mg/dl; sodium: 115 mg; total carbohydrate: 16 g; dietary fiber: 2 g; sugar: 10 g; protein: 5 g; vitamin A: 0 mcg; vitamin C: 0 mg; calcium: 26 mg; iron: 0.7 mg

Rich in vitamin E, niacin, copper, and manganese

No-Bake Peanut Butter Oat Bars

MAKES 10 BARS
MILK MAKER: oats
SUPERFOODS: almonds, peanuts

1 cup (160 g) pitted Medjool dates
1½ cups (120 g) rolled oats
1 cup (120 g) chopped roasted almonds
¼ cup (60 g) mini chocolate chips, optional

¼ cup (60 ml) agave nectar
¼ cup (65 g) creamy peanut butter
½ teaspoon vanilla extract

1. Line an 8-inch (20 cm) square baking dish with parchment paper.

2. Process the dates in a food processor until a sticky paste forms. Scrape the date paste into a large bowl and add the oats and almonds. Stir in the chocolate chips, if using. Using your hands or a sturdy spoon, mix to combine.

3. Warm the agave nectar, peanut butter, and vanilla extract in a small sauce-pan over low heat until the peanut butter has melted and all the ingredients have completely combined. Stir and pour over the oat mixture. Stir together until all of the components are evenly disturbed.

4. Transfer to the prepared baking dish, pressing to flatten the mixture evenly.

5. Cover and refrigerate for at least 20 minutes to harden. Remove the bars from the pan by lifting out the parchment paper and cut into ten even bars. Store in an airtight container for up to a 4 days. The bars can also be frozen if you don't plan on eating them all within 3 to 4 days.

PER BAR Calories: 270; total fat: 13 g; saturated fat: 2.5 g; cholesterol: 0 mg/dl; sodium: 0 mg; total carbohydrate: 34 g; dietary fiber: 5 g; sugar: 21 g; protein: 7 g; vitamin A: 0 mcg; vitamin C: 0 mg; calcium: 52 mg; iron: 1.8 mg
Rich in iron, vitamin E, riboflavin, niacin, magnesium, copper, and manganese

Chocolate Malt Superfood Bars

MAKES 20 BARS
MILK MAKER: barley malt
SUPERFOODS: chia seeds, hemp seeds, pecans, walnuts, almonds

BARS

½ cup (80 g) pitted Medjool dates

½ cup (60 g) raw walnut halves

¼ cup (35 g) whole, raw almonds

3 tablespoons unsweetened cocoa
 powder

2 tablespoons barley malt syrup

2 tablespoons chia seeds

2 tablespoons coconut oil

2 tablespoons organic raw, shelled
 hemp seeds

TOPPINGS

¼ cup (65 g) almond butter

¼ cup (40 g) pitted Medjool dates

2 tablespoons barley malt syrup

2 tablespoons tahini

1 teaspoon vanilla extract

¾ cup (80 g) chopped pecans

CHOCOLATE MALT SAUCE

3 tablespoons coconut oil

3 tablespoons unsweetened cocoa
 powder

2 tablespoons agave nectar

1 tablespoons barley malt syrup

RECIPE CONTINUES →

1. Line an 8-inch (20 cm) square baking dish with parchment paper.

2. To make the Bars, combine all of the bar ingredients in a food processor and process into a crumbly dough. Transfer to the prepared baking dish, pressing to flatten the mixture evenly. Place the baking dish in the freezer while working on the toppings.

3. To make the Toppings, place the almond butter, dates, malt syrup, tahini, and vanilla in a food processor and process until smooth. Remove the bar base from the freezer and spread the topping over the base. Top with ½ cup (55 g) of the chopped pecans, then return to the freezer.

4. To make the Chocolate Malt Sauce, melt the coconut oil in a small saucepan over low heat. Whisk in the cocoa powder, agave, and malt syrup. Whisk until smooth.

5. Pour the Chocolate Malt Sauce over the bars, sprinkle with the last ¼ cup (25 g) of the pecans, return to the freezer, and allow to set for about 4 hours.

PER BAR Calories: 170; total fat: 13 g; saturated fat: 4 g; cholesterol: 0 mg/dl; sodium: 0 mg; total carbohydrate: 13 g; dietary fiber: 3 g; sugar: 10 g; protein: 3 g; vitamin A: 0 mcg; vitamin C: 0 mg; calcium: 52 mg; iron: 1.1 mg
Rich in magnesium, copper, and manganese

Falafel Roasted Chickpeas

MAKES 1½ CUPS (250 G)
SUPERFOOD: chickpeas

1½ cups (250 g) cooked chickpeas
1 tablespoon olive oil
¾ teaspoon cumin
½ teaspoon garlic powder
½ teaspoon paprika
½ teaspoon onion powder
¼ teaspoon ground coriander
⅛ teaspoon salt

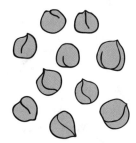

1. Preheat the oven to 400°F (200°C). Line a baking sheet with parchment paper.

2. Toss the chickpeas with the olive oil, cumin, garlic powder, paprika, onion powder, coriander, and salt in a medium bowl, evenly coating all the chickpeas. Spread in an even layer on the prepared baking sheet and roast for 30 to 40 minutes, until golden brown and crispy. Midway through the baking, stir the chickpeas.

3. Remove from the oven and allow to cool to room temperature before serving.

PER SERVING (ABOUT ⅓ CUP/55 G; 4 SERVINGS PER RECIPE) Calories: 140; total fat: 5 g; saturated fat: 0.5 g; cholesterol: 0 mg/dl; sodium: 70mg; total carbohydrate: 18 g; dietary fiber: 5 g; sugar: 3 g; protein: 6 g; vitamin A: 54 mcg; vitamin C: 2 mg; calcium: 26 mg; iron: 1.8 mg
Rich in iron, folate, manganese, and copper

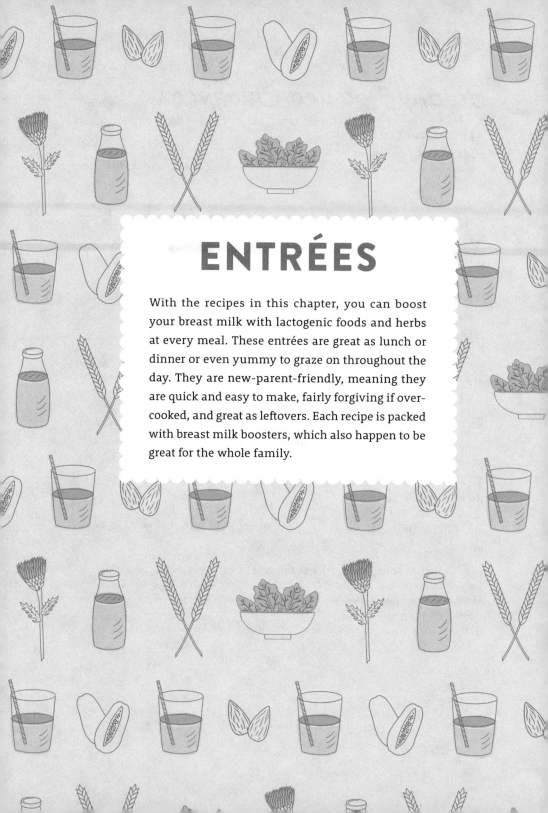

ENTRÉES

With the recipes in this chapter, you can boost your breast milk with lactogenic foods and herbs at every meal. These entrées are great as lunch or dinner or even yummy to graze on throughout the day. They are new-parent-friendly, meaning they are quick and easy to make, fairly forgiving if overcooked, and great as leftovers. Each recipe is packed with breast milk boosters, which also happen to be great for the whole family.

Creamy Barley Risotto

MAKES 4 SERVINGS
MILK MAKER: barley
SUPERFOODS: carrots, chickpeas

3 cups (720 ml) vegetable broth
1 cup (200 g) pearl barley
¼ cup (35 g) cubed fresh butternut squash
1 medium carrot, sliced into ¼-inch (6 mm) medallions
1 tablespoon extra virgin olive oil
¼ cup (40 g) cooked chickpeas
¼ cup (60 ml) milk of choice
1 garlic clove, minced
Pinch plus ¼ teaspoon salt

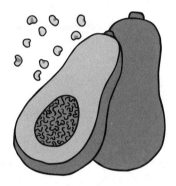

1. Combine the broth and barley in a medium stockpot and bring to a boil. Reduce the heat to medium-low and simmer uncovered for 40 minutes. Turn the heat to low, cover, and cook for an additional 10 minutes. Remove from the heat and fluff with a fork.

2. Preheat the oven to 425°F (220°C). Line a baking sheet with parchment paper. Toss the butternut squash and carrot in the oil. Sprinkle with a pinch of salt and roast for 15 to 20 minutes, until tender.

3. Blend the roasted vegetables, chickpeas, milk, garlic, and remaining salt in a blender or food processor until smooth. Pour the sauce over the barley and stir to coat. Serve warm.

PER SERVING Calories: 250; total fat: 5 g; saturated fat: 0.5 g; cholesterol: 0 mg/dl; sodium: 870 mg; total carbohydrate: 48 g; dietary fiber: 9 g; sugar: 4 g; protein: 7 g; vitamin A: 1,170 mcg; vitamin C: 4 mg; calcium: 26 mg; iron: 1.8 mg

Rich in iron, potassium, vitamin A, thiamin, vitamin B6, niacin, phosphorous, magnesium, zinc, selenium, copper, and manganese

Slow-Cooked White Bean Chili

MAKES 4 SERVINGS
SUPERFOOD: cannellini beans

6 cups (1.4 L) low-sodium vegetable broth

2 cups (360 g) dried cannellini beans

One 14.5-ounce (410 g) can diced fire-roasted tomatoes

½ bell pepper, diced

½ medium onion, diced

4 garlic cloves, minced

2 teaspoons chili powder

2 teaspoons ground cumin

2 teaspoons dried oregano

1 teaspoon salt, or to taste

¼ teaspoon white pepper

Combine all the ingredients in a slow cooker. Cover and cook on low for at least 8 hours. Serve warm.

PER SERVING Calories: 380; total fat: 0.5 g; saturated fat: 0 g; cholesterol: 0 mg/dl; sodium: 1,160 mg; total carbohydrate: 68 g; dietary fiber: 18 g; sugar: 12 g; protein: 25 g; vitamin A: 450 mcg; vitamin C: 36 mg; calcium: 325 mg; iron: 10.8 mg
Rich in calcium, iron, vitamin A, and vitamin C

Beluga Lentil Burgers

MAKE 7 BURGERS
SUPERFOOD: lentils

1½ cups (390 g) cooked beluga lentils

1 tablespoon Bragg liquid aminos

1 tablespoon extra virgin olive oil

1 teaspoon smoked paprika

1 teaspoon vegan Worcestershire sauce

½ teaspoon onion powder

¼ teaspoon garlic powder

⅛ teaspoon dried thyme

⅓ cup (40 g) vital wheat gluten

Oil for the pan

7 hamburger buns

4 leaves of romaine lettuce, cut in half

Optional toppings: Bread and butter pickles, tomato slices, ketchup, and mustard

1. Combine the lentils, liquid aminos, olive oil, paprika, Worcestershire sauce, onion powder, garlic powder, and thyme in a medium bowl. Mash the lentils with the back of a wooden spoon until a little over half of the lentils are mashed. Stir in the wheat gluten and continue to mash until completely incorporated. Divide the lentils into seven balls and flatten into patties about ⅛ inch (3 mm) thick.

2. Add enough oil to lightly cover the bottom of a heavy-bottomed pan like a cast-iron skillet and warm the oil over medium heat. Cook three or four patties at a time, cooking until lightly brown on both sides (3 to 5 minutes per side). Assemble the burgers on the buns with toppings and enjoy.

PER BURGER Calories: 290; total fat: 6 g; saturated fat: 1 g; cholesterol: 0 mg/dl; sodium: 540 mg; total carbohydrate: 47 g; dietary fiber: 6 g; sugar: 7 g; protein: 16 g; vitamin A: 1,170 mcg; vitamin C: 2 mg; calcium: 52 mg; iron: 3.6 mg
Rich in iron, vitamin A, vitamin K, thiamin, riboflavin, niacin, and folate

Impossibly Good Curry

MAKES 4 SERVINGS
MILK MAKER: fenugreek seeds
SUPERFOOD: tofu

14 ounces (400 g) extra firm tofu, pressed and cubed

6 whole cardamom pods

6 whole cloves

10 whole peppercorns, any color

2 teaspoons fenugreek seeds

3 tablespoons extra virgin olive oil

½ medium onion, diced

3 garlic cloves, sliced thin

3 bay leaves

1 cinnamon stick

1-inch (2.5 cm) piece fresh ginger, minced or grated

3 tablespoons curry powder

1½ tablespoons brown sugar

½ teaspoon ground coriander

¼ teaspoon red pepper flakes, optional

1½ cups (360 ml) water

½ cup (120 ml) coconut milk

1 tablespoon fresh lemon juice

⅛ teaspoon salt

RECIPE CONTINUES →

1. Preheat the oven to 425°F (220°C). Line a baking sheet with parchment paper.

2. Place the cubed tofu in a single layer on the prepared baking sheet and bake about 15 to 20 minutes, until firm. While the tofu is roasting, prepare the curry.

3. Place the cardamom, cloves, peppercorns, and fenugreek seeds in the center of a 5-inch (13 cm) square piece of cheesecloth and tie closed in a bouquet garni, making sure that the contents can't easily escape.

4. Warm the oil in a medium saucepan over medium heat and cook the onion until lightly browned, 3 to 5 minutes. Add the garlic and cook until tender, about 1 minute. Mix in the bay leaves, cinnamon stick, ginger, curry powder, brown sugar, coriander, and red pepper flakes, if using. Cook and stir for about 3 minutes. Pour in the water and bring to a boil. Add the bouquet garni. Reduce the heat to low, cover, and simmer for 30 minutes.

5. Mix in the coconut milk, lemon juice, salt, and roasted tofu and continue cooking for at least 15 minutes. Remove the bouquet garni, cinnamon stick, and bay leaves before serving.

PER SERVING Calories: 300; total fat: 23 g; saturated fat: 6 g; cholesterol: 0 mg; sodium: 95 mg; total carbohydrate: 17 g; dietary fiber: 6 g; sugar: 6 g; protein: 12 g; vitamin A: 18 mcg; vitamin C: 5 mg; calcium: 260 mg; iron: 4.5 mg
Rich in calcium, iron, pantothenic acid, phosphorus, magnesium, zinc, selenium, copper, and manganese

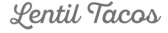

Lentil Tacos

MAKES 12 TACOS
SUPERFOODS: lentils, avocado

1 tablespoon canola oil

½ small sweet onion, diced

1 garlic clove, minced

⅔ cup (125 g) dried lentils, rinsed and picked over

1 tablespoon Taco Seasoning (page 178)

1⅔ cups (400 ml) vegetable broth

12 small whole wheat flour tortillas, corn tortillas, or crispy tacos shells

1 batch New Mom Guacamole (page 191), or 1 avocado, peeled, pitted, and sliced thin

1. Warm the oil in a small saucepan over medium heat. Add the onion and cook until translucent, about 5 minutes. Add the garlic and cook until fragrant, about 1 minute. Add the lentils and Taco Seasoning and stir to coat. Add the vegetable broth and bring to a boil.

2. Reduce the heat to low, cover the pan, and simmer until the lentils are tender, about 25 minutes. Uncover the pan and continue to cook on low until most of the liquid has been absorbed. Divide the lentils among the tortillas, top with guacamole or sliced avocado, and serve.

PER TACO Calories: 150; total fat: 6 g; saturated fat: 0.5 g; cholesterol: 0 mg/dl; sodium: 280 mg; total carbohydrate: 21 g; dietary fiber: 7 g; sugar: 2 g; protein: 5 g; vitamin A: 72 mcg; vitamin C: 4 mg; calcium: 26 mg; iron: 1.4 mg
Rich in thiamin, vitamin B6, folate, pantothenic acid, phosphorus, magnesium, zinc, copper, and manganese

Teriyaki Portobello Steaks

MAKES 4 SERVINGS
MILK MAKER: mushrooms

1 pound (455 g) portobello mushrooms (about 4 large caps; see Note)
½ cup (120 ml) Bragg liquid aminos
½ cup (120 ml) canola oil
⅓ cup (80 ml) white vinegar
¼ cup (60 ml) agave nectar
2 to 4 tablespoons minced fresh ginger or ginger juice
4 garlic cloves, sliced thin

1. Clean the mushrooms by rubbing a wet cloth over the caps. Whisk together the remaining ingredients in a bowl to make a marinade.

RECIPE CONTINUES →

2. Place the mushrooms in a large ziplock bag and add the marinade. Close the bag tightly and marinate for at least an hour but up to 24 hours for maximum flavor.

3. Preheat the oven to 425°F (220°C). Line a rimmed baking sheet with foil. Bake the marinated mushrooms on the bottom rack of the oven for 15 to 20 minutes, until the mushrooms are tender.

NOTE: You can use 1 pound (455 g) cremini mushrooms in place of the portobello mushrooms.

PER STEAK Calories: 120; total fat: 7 g; saturated fat: 0.5 g; cholesterol: 0 mg/dl; sodium: 490 mg; total carbohydrate: 13 g; dietary fiber: 2 g; sugar: 10 g; protein: 3 g; vitamin A: 0 mcg; vitamin C: 0 mg; calcium: 0 mg; iron: 0.4 mg
Rich in riboflavin, niacin, vitamin B6, pantothenic acid, phosphorus, selenium, and copper

Chia-Flecked Empanadas

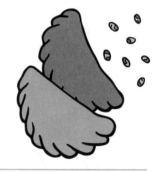

MAKES 24 EMPANADAS
MILK MAKERS: whole wheat pastry flour
SUPERFOODS: chia seeds, pinto beans

EMPANADA DOUGH

¼ cup (60 ml) water

1 tablespoon ground or whole chia seeds

1¼ cups (150 g) whole wheat pastry flour

1 cup (125 g) all-purpose flour

½ cup (115 g) Earth Balance margarine or trans-fat-free vegetable shortening, cut into cubes

1 teaspoon salt

⅓ cup (80 ml) ice water

1 tablespoon white vinegar

Oil for baking

FILLING

1½ cups (255 g) cooked pinto beans	1 teaspoon Taco Seasoning (page 178)
⅓ cup (80 ml) salsa	⅛ teaspoon salt

1. **To make the Empanada Dough,** whisk together the water and chia seeds in a small bowl; set aside.

2. Combine the whole wheat pastry flour, all-purpose flour, margarine, and salt in a large bowl with a fork or handheld pastry blender until the mixture resembles coarse cornmeal.

3. Add the chia mixture, ice water, and vinegar, stirring with a fork until combined.

4. Turn out the mixture onto a lightly floured surface and knead gently to bring the dough together. Form the dough into a flat rectangle and chill, wrapped in plastic wrap, for at least 1 hour.

5. **To make the Filling,** combine all the ingredients in a small bowl; set aside.

6. Preheat the oven to 400°F (200°C).

7. Roll out the dough to ⅛ inch (3 mm) thick and cut into small 3-inch (7.5 cm) circles. Place 1 tablespoon of the filling into each empanada square, fold it over, and seal by pressing the edges together. Brush the empanadas with oil and bake for 15 to 20 minutes, until puffed slightly and golden brown.

PER SERVING (4 EMPANADAS) Calories: 370; total fat: 16 g; saturated fat: 4 g; cholesterol: 0 mg/dl; sodium: 630 mg; total carbohydrate: 47 g; dietary fiber: 9 g; sugar: <1 g; protein: 9 g; vitamin A: 36 mcg; vitamin C: 0 mg; calcium: 26 mg; iron: 2.7 mg
Rich in iron, vitamin E, thiamin, riboflavin, folate, selenium, copper, and manganese

Lentil Fritters

MAKES 20 FRITTERS
SUPERFOODS: chia seeds, lentils

½ cup (120 ml) water

2 tablespoons ground chia seeds

3 cups (600 g) cooked lentils

½ cup (10 g) chopped fresh cilantro

2 tablespoons chopped fresh
  flat-leaf parsley

1 garlic clove, minced

½ teaspoon ground cumin

½ cup (60 g) plain bread crumbs

½ teaspoon salt

¼ teaspoon black pepper

2 tablespoons olive oil

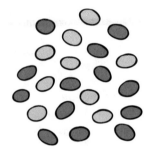

1. Whisk together the water and chia seeds and set aside.

2. In a food processor, puree 1½ cups (300 g) of the lentils with the cilantro, parsley, garlic, and cumin until nearly smooth. Transfer to a bowl and mix in the bread crumbs, chia mixture, the remaining lentils, salt, and pepper. Form into twenty patties about ½ inch (13 mm) thick (about 2 tablespoons each).

3. Heat 1 tablespoon of the oil in a large nonstick skillet over medium-high heat. Working in two batches, cook the patties until browned, 3 to 4 minutes per side, adding the remaining tablespoon of oil to the skillet for the second batch.

PER FRITTER Calories: 60; total fat: 2 g; saturated fat: 0 g; cholesterol: 0 mg/dl; sodium: 80 mg; total carbohydrate: 8 g; dietary fiber: 3 g; sugar: <1 g; protein: 3 g; vitamin A: 18 mcg; vitamin C: 2 mg; calcium: 26 mg; iron: 1.4 mg
Rich in folate and copper

Lentil Samosas

MAKES 30 SAMOSAS
MILK MAKER: whole wheat pastry flour
SUPERFOODS: lentils, carrots, turmeric

DOUGH

1½ cups (180 g) whole wheat pastry flour

1 cup (125 g) all-purpose flour

1 cup (225 g) Earth Balance margarine

½ teaspoon salt

¼ to ½ cup (60 to 120 ml) cold water

FILLING

3 cups (720 ml) water, plus more if needed

1 cup (200 g) dried lentils

2 tablespoons olive oil

½ medium onion, diced

2 medium potatoes, scrubbed and diced

1 yellow bell pepper, seeded and diced

1 large carrot, peeled and diced

5 garlic cloves, minced

2-inch (5 cm) piece fresh ginger, minced

2 teaspoons curry powder

1½ teaspoons garam masala

1 teaspoon chili powder

1 teaspoon ground cumin

1 teaspoon ground turmeric

1 teaspoon paprika

½ teaspoon salt

1. To make the Dough, process the flours, ½ cup (115 g) of the margarine, and the salt in a food processor until the mixture resembles coarse cornmeal. Add the remaining ½ cup (115 g) margarine and pulse five more times to combine. With the machine running, slowly pour in just enough water to form a dough. Divide the dough in half and press gently into two disks. Wrap each disk in plastic wrap and refrigerate for at least 30 minutes or up to 8 hours.

2. To make the Filling, pour the water and lentils into a medium saucepan and bring to a boil. Cover, reduce the heat to medium-low, and simmer until the lentils are tender, 20 to 25 minutes.

RECIPE CONTINUES →

3. While the lentils are cooking, warm the oil in a medium stockpot over medium heat. Add the onion and cook until translucent, about 5 minutes. Add the potatoes, bell pepper, carrot, garlic, ginger, curry powder, garam masala, chili powder, cumin, turmeric, paprika, and salt. Cook for 10 minutes, stirring frequently. Add additional water 1 tablespoon at a time if the mixture begins to dry out and stick to the pot.

4. Stir in the cooked lentils and cook for 10 minutes, stirring and adding water as needed.

5. Preheat the oven to 375°F (190°C). Line a large baking sheet with parchment paper.

6. Remove one disk of dough from the refrigerator and roll out to ⅛-inch (3 mm) thickness on a smooth, well-floured surface. Cut into 3-inch (7.5 cm) circles with a biscuit or cookie cutter. Add 1 rounded tablespoon of filling to each circle and fold in half. Seal the edges with the tines of a fork. Arrange the samosas in a single layer close to each other on the prepared baking sheet. Bake for 15 to 20 minutes, until golden brown.

PER SAMOSA Calories: 140; total fat: 7 g; saturated fat: 2 g; cholesterol: 0 mg/dl; sodium: 140 mg; total carbohydrate: 15 g; dietary fiber: 3 g; sugar: 0 g; protein: 3 g; vitamin A: 135 mcg; vitamin C: 14 mg; calcium: 0 mg; iron: 1.1 mg
Rich in vitamin A, vitamin C, and folate

Green Papaya Pad Thai

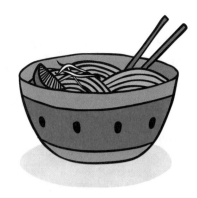

MAKES 2 SERVINGS

MILK MAKER: green papaya

SUPERFOODS: peanuts, tofu

3 tablespoons Bragg liquid aminos

3 tablespoons sugar

1 tablespoon tamarind paste

¼ cup (60 ml) canola oil

14 ounces (400 g) firm tofu, cubed

3 small garlic cloves, sliced thin

1 small shallot, sliced thin

1½ cups (210 g) shredded green papaya

1 cup (105 g) bean sprouts, washed and dried

½ cup (75 g) chopped roasted peanuts

Lime wedges

1. Combine the liquid aminos, sugar, and tamarind paste in a small saucepan. Cook over medium heat until the mixture reaches a low boil. Give the sauce a good stir, remove from the heat, and set aside.

2. Warm 2 tablespoons of the oil in a large frying pan or wok. Sauté the tofu until lightly brown and crispy, 4 to 5 minutes. Remove the tofu from the pan and set aside in a small bowl.

3. Heat the remaining 2 tablespoons oil in the pan over medium-high heat. Add the garlic and shallot to the hot pan and cook for 1 minute, stirring constantly with a wok spatula or large wooden spoon. Add the cooked tofu.

4. Add the shredded papaya and stir to incorporate. Add the sauce, stirring constantly until the mixture is well coated. Divide between two plates and top with the bean sprouts and peanuts. Garnish with the lime wedges.

PER SERVING Calories: 960; total fat: 65 g; saturated fat: 7 g; cholesterol: 0 mg/dl; sodium: 1,490 mg; total carbohydrate: 68 g; dietary fiber: 13 g; sugar: 40 g; protein: 46 g; vitamin A: 1,050 mcg; vitamin C: 108 mg; calcium: 1,430 mg; iron: 7.2 mg

Rich in vitamin A, vitamin C, calcium, iron, vitamin E, vitamin K, thiamin, riboflavin, niacin, vitamin B6, folate, pantothenic acid, phosphorus, magnesium, zinc, selenium, copper, and manganese

Moringa Poricha Kootu

MAKES 2 SERVINGS
MILK MAKER: moringa
SUPERFOODS: yellow split peas, turmeric

¾ cup (180 ml) water
¼ cup (50 g) dried yellow split peas, soaked for at least 1 hour
1 cup (30 g) packed fresh moringa leaves
1 teaspoon ground turmeric
¼ cup (60 ml) coconut milk
1 teaspoon urad dal (black gram), optional
½ teaspoon sambar powder
½ teaspoon whole cumin seeds
½ teaspoon whole yellow mustard seeds
¼ teaspoon salt

1. Combine the water and split peas in a medium stockpot and bring to a boil. Reduce the heat to medium-low and cook until tender and thickened, 15 to 20 minutes. Add more water, if necessary, to prevent drying out.

2. Stir in the moringa leaves and turmeric and cook for an additional 15 minutes, or until the leaves are tender. Add the coconut milk, urad dal, if using, sambar, cumin seeds, mustard seeds, and salt to the pot and cook for an additional 5 minutes. Serve warm, preferably over rice.

PER SERVING Calories: 130; total fat: 6 g; saturated fat: 3.5 g; cholesterol: 0 mg/dl; sodium: 310 mg; total carbohydrate: 18 g; dietary fiber: 7 g; sugar: 1 g; protein: 8 g; vitamin A: 180 mcg; vitamin C: 23 mg; calcium: 104 mg; iron: 3.6 mg
Rich in calcium, iron, vitamin A, vitamin C, vitamin E, vitamin K, vitamin B6, and manganese

Gnocchi with Moringa Pesto

MAKES 6 SERVINGS
MILK MAKER: moringa
SUPERFOODS: basil, pine nuts

1½ ounces (45 g) fresh basil leaves

½ cup (120 ml) extra virgin olive oil

½ cup (70 g) pine nuts

2 garlic cloves, peeled

1 tablespoon nutritional yeast

1 tablespoon plus 1 teaspoon moringa powder

¼ teaspoon salt

1 pound (455 g) gnocchi, cooked according to package directions

Combine all the ingredients except the gnocchi in a food processor and process until smooth. Toss with the gnocchi and serve warm.

PER SERVING Calories: 370; total fat: 27 g; saturated fat: 3 g; cholesterol: <5 mg/dl; sodium: 480 mg; total carbohydrate: 28 g; dietary fiber: 2 g; sugar: 4 g; protein: 7 g; vitamin A: 135 mcg; vitamin C: 14 mg; calcium: 52 mg; iron: 1.8 mg
Rich in iron, potassium, vitamin A, vitamin C, vitamin K, copper, and manganese

Roasted Balsamic Tempeh

MAKES 4 SERVINGS
SUPERFOOD: tempeh

½ cup (120 ml) balsamic vinegar
3 tablespoons extra virgin olive oil
2 tablespoons Bragg liquid aminos
2 tablespoons maple syrup
1 teaspoon dried thyme
¼ teaspoon garlic powder
8 ounces (225 g) tempeh, cubed

1. Whisk together the vinegar, olive oil, liquid aminos, maple syrup, thyme, and garlic powder in an 8-inch (20 cm) square baking dish. Add the tempeh and stir to coat. Cover and marinate for 8 to 24 hours.

2. Preheat the oven to 375°F (190°C). Uncover the tempeh and place the baking dish in the oven. Bake for 30 to 40 minutes, until the tempeh is tender and the majority of the marinade has been absorbed.

PER SERVING Calories: 250; total fat: 17 g; saturated fat: 2.5 g; cholesterol: 0 mg/dl; sodium: 490 mg; total carbohydrate: 18 g; dietary fiber: 4 g; sugar: 13 g; protein: 12 g; vitamin A: 0 mcg; vitamin C: 0 mg; calcium: 78 mg; iron: 1.8 mg
Rich in iron, riboflavin, niacin, phosphorus, magnesium, copper, and manganese

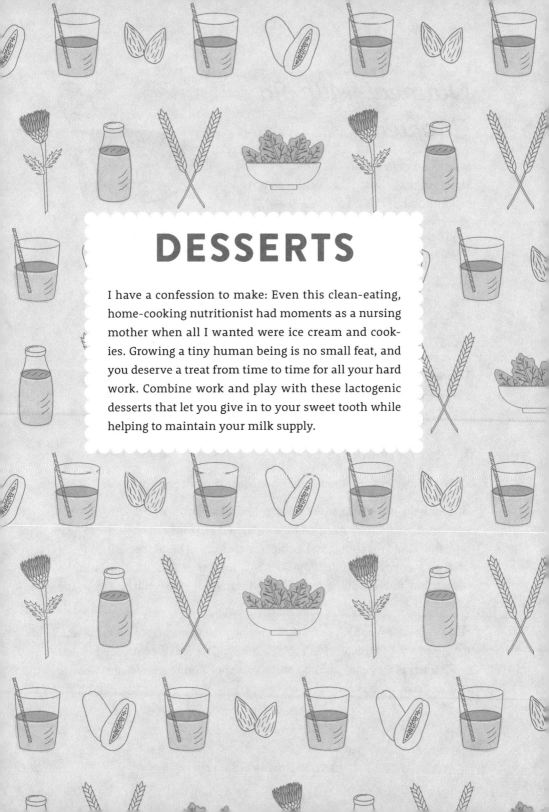

DESSERTS

I have a confession to make: Even this clean-eating, home-cooking nutritionist had moments as a nursing mother when all I wanted were ice cream and cookies. Growing a tiny human being is no small feat, and you deserve a treat from time to time for all your hard work. Combine work and play with these lactogenic desserts that let you give in to your sweet tooth while helping to maintain your milk supply.

Oatmeal Milk-In Cookies

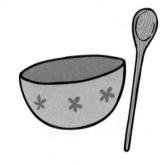

MAKES 40 COOKIES
MILK MAKERS: barley, oats, whole wheat flour
SUPERFOODS: chia seeds, hemp seeds

½ cup (120 ml) water or barley water (page 146)

2 tablespoons ground chia seeds

¾ cup (150 g) granulated sugar

¾ cup (165 g) packed light brown sugar

¾ cup (170 g) Earth Balance margarine, softened

1 teaspoon vanilla extract

1 teaspoon baking soda

½ teaspoon ground cinnamon

½ teaspoon cream of tartar

½ teaspoon salt

1¼ cups (150 g) whole wheat pastry flour

1¾ cups (140 g) rolled oats

1 cup (90 g) barley flakes

¼ cup plus 2 tablespoons (60 g) organic raw, shelled hemp seeds

½ cup (72.5 g) raisins

1. Preheat the oven to 375°F (190°C).

2. Whisk together the water and chia seeds in a small bowl, set aside.

3. Cream the granulated sugar, brown sugar, margarine, and vanilla in a large bowl with an electric mixer. Add the chia seed mixture and continue to beat until fluffy. Add the baking soda, cinnamon, cream of tartar, and salt and beat until incorporated. Add the flour and beat until incorporated. Then add the oats, barley flakes, and hemp seeds and mix until incorporated. Stir in the raisins.

4. Using a tablespoon measure, drop the dough onto ungreased cookie sheets. Bake for 10 to 13 minutes, until golden brown. The cookies will look soft but will harden as they cool. Cool slightly on the sheets and then transfer to a wire rack and cool completely.

Ginger Chia Seed Cookies

MAKES 12 COOKIES
MILK MAKER: oats
SUPERFOOD: chia seeds

3 tablespoons milk of choice

1 tablespoon whole chia seeds, plus more for sprinkling

1 cup (80 g) rolled oats

¼ cup (50 g) sugar

½ teaspoon baking soda

¼ teaspoon baking powder

⅛ teaspoon salt

1 tablespoon freshly grated ginger or ginger juice

1 tablespoon maple syrup

½ teaspoon vanilla extract

¼ cup (60 g) Earth Balance margarine

1. Preheat the oven to 350°F (180°C). Line a baking sheet with parchment paper.

2. Combine the milk and chia seeds in a small bowl and set aside for at least 10 minutes.

3. Blend the oats in a food processor until you have a coarse flour. Add the sugar, baking soda, baking powder, and salt and pulse just to mix. Add the ginger, maple syrup, vanilla, margarine, and the chia seed mixture and pulse until the dough starts to form a ball.

4. Remove the dough from the food processor and form into a ball. Wrap in plastic wrap and refrigerate for up to 24 hours. Roll out the dough to ¼ inch (6 mm) thick. Using a cookie cutter, cut out circles and place on the prepared baking sheet. Sprinkle the tops with chia seeds.

RECIPE CONTINUES →

5. Bake for 15 to 18 minutes, until the cookies are golden brown. Allow to cool completely before eating.

PER COOKIE Calories: 90; total fat: 4.5 g; saturated fat: 1 g; cholesterol: 0 mg/dl; sodium: 110 mg; total carbohydrate: 10 g; dietary fiber: 1 g; sugar: 6 g; protein: 1 g; vitamin A: 0 mcg; vitamin C: 0 mg; calcium: 0 mg; iron: 0.4 mg

Almond-Lime Shortbread

MAKES 24 COOKIES
SUPERFOOD: almonds

2 cups (220 g) almond flour
⅓ cup (70 g) sugar
¼ cup plus 2 tablespoons (85 g) Earth Balance margarine, melted
1 tablespoon grated lime zest

1. Stir the almond flour, sugar, margarine, and zest in a large bowl until combined into a dough. Shape the dough into a 6-inch (15 cm) log and wrap tightly in plastic wrap. Refrigerate for at least 30 minutes or overnight.

2. Preheat the oven to 350°F (180°C) and line a baking sheet with parchment paper.

3. Slice the dough into ¼-inch (6 mm) circles or squares and place on the prepared baking sheet close together; they won't expand while baking. Bake for 10 to 15 minutes, until golden brown and firm. Allow to cool completely before removing from the pan.

PER COOKIE Calories: 90; total fat: 7 g; saturated fat: 1 g; cholesterol: 0 mg/dl; sodium: 30 mg; total carbohydrate: 5 g; dietary fiber: 1 g; sugar: 3 g; protein: 2 g; vitamin A: 0 mcg; vitamin C: 2 mg; calcium: 26 mg; iron: 0.4 mg

Peanut Butter Malted Cookies

MAKES 24 COOKIES

MILK MAKER: barley malt, whole wheat pastry flour
SUPERFOODS: chia seeds, peanut butter

½ cup (120 ml) water

2 tablespoons ground chia seeds

1 cup (335 g) barley malt syrup

1 cup (260 g) peanut butter

1 cup (225 g) Earth Balance
margarine, softened

¼ cup (55 g) packed brown sugar

½ cup (100 g) granulated sugar

1½ teaspoons baking soda

1 teaspoon baking powder

½ teaspoon salt

2½ cups (300 g) whole wheat pastry
flour

1. Whisk together the water and chia seeds in a small bowl; set aside.

2. Beat the barley malt syrup, peanut butter, margarine, brown sugar, and granulated sugar together in a bowl using an electric mixer until smooth and creamy. Add the chia seed mixture and beat until smooth.

3. Add the baking soda, baking powder, and salt and beat to incorporate. Add the flour and beat until a soft dough forms. Cover the bowl and refrigerate for at least 1 hour or overnight.

4. Preheat the oven to 375°F (190°C). Line a large baking sheet with parchment paper.

5. Roll the dough into 1-inch (2.5 cm) balls and arrange on the baking sheet 2 inches (5 cm) apart. Flatten each ball using a fork, making a crisscross pattern.

6. Bake for 7 to 10 minutes, until golden brown, making sure not to overbake.

PER COOKIE Calories: 260; total fat: 13 g; saturated fat: 3 g; cholesterol: 0 mg/dl; sodium: 250 mg; total carbohydrate: 30 g; dietary fiber: 3 g; sugar: 19 g; protein: 5 g; vitamin A: 0 mcg; vitamin C: 0 mg; calcium: 26 mg; iron: 0.7 mg
Rich in niacin and copper

Almond Butter Cookies

MAKES 16 COOKIES
MILK MAKER: oats
SUPERFOODS: almonds, chia seeds

¼ cup (60 ml) water

1 tablespoon ground chia seeds

¾ cup (190 g) almond butter

½ cup (115 g) Earth Balance margarine, softened

¾ cup (165 g) packed dark brown sugar

2 tablespoons maple syrup

1 teaspoon vanilla extract

1½ cups (160 g) oat flour (see page 135)

1 teaspoon baking soda

½ teaspoon salt

1. Whisk together the water and chia seeds in a small bowl; set aside.

2. Cream the almond butter and margarine using an electric mixer until fluffy. Add the sugar and maple syrup and beat on high for about 2 minutes, scraping down the sides of the bowl as necessary. Reduce the speed to medium and add the chia mixture and vanilla; beat until well blended. Add the oat flour, baking soda, and salt and beat until just combined. Cover and place the bowl in the fridge for at least 30 minutes or up to 24 hours.

3. Preheat the oven to 350°F (180°C) and line two baking sheets with parchment paper.

3. Scoop out a rounded tablespoon of dough and roll to form a ball. Place the balls on the baking sheets about 2 inches apart. With a fork dipped lightly in oat flour, press the tines onto the dough to lightly flatten in a crisscross pattern.

4. Bake for 9 to 11 minutes, until the cookies are lightly browned and just set. Remove from the oven and let cool 2 minutes on the baking sheets.

PER COOKIE Calories: 260; total fat: 13 g; saturated fat: 3 g; cholesterol: 0 mg/dl; sodium: 250 mg; total carbohydrate: 30 g; dietary fiber: 3 g; sugar: 19 g; protein: 5 g; vitamin A: 0 mcg; vitamin C: 0 mg; calcium: 26 mg; iron: 0.7 mg
Rich in niacin and copper

Snickerdoodles

MAKES 24 COOKIES

SUPERFOODS: chia seeds, almonds

½ cup (120 ml) water

2 tablespoons ground chia seeds

½ cup (115 g) Earth Balance margarine, softened

½ cup (100 g) granulated sugar

¼ cup (55 g) packed light brown sugar

¼ cup (60 g) nonhydrogenated vegetable shortening

1 teaspoon vanilla extract

½ teaspoon baking soda

½ teaspoon ground cinnamon

½ teaspoon salt

3 cups plus 3 tablespoons (350 g) almond flour

TOPPING

¼ cup (50 g) granulated sugar

1½ teaspoons ground cinnamon

1. Preheat the oven to 350°F (180°C). Line a large baking sheet with parchment paper.

2. Whisk together the water and chia seeds in a small bowl; set aside.

3. Cream the margarine, sugars, and shortening together with an electric mixer. Add the vanilla, baking soda, cinnamon, salt, and chia seed mixture together and beat until combined. Add the almond flour, 1 cup (110 g) at a time, until completely incorporated.

4. To make the topping, stir together the sugar and cinnamon in a small bowl. One rounded tablespoon at a time, roll the cookie dough into a ball and then roll to coat in the sugar-cinnamon mixture. Place the coated balls on the prepared baking sheet about 2 inches (5 cm) apart. They will spread substantially while baking.

RECIPE CONTINUES →

5. Bake for 10 to 12 minutes, until golden brown. Cool on the baking sheet to room temperature. The cookies can be stored in an airtight container for up to a week. They also freeze well.

PER COOKIE Calories: 170; total fat: 14 g; saturated fat: 2.5 g; cholesterol: 0 mg/dl; sodium: 115 mg; total carbohydrate: 11 g; dietary fiber: 2 g; sugar: 8 g; protein: 3 g; vitamin A: 0 mcg; vitamin C: 0 mg; calcium: 52 mg; iron: 0.7 mg
Rich in vitamin E and magnesium

Cinnamon Cardamom Blondies

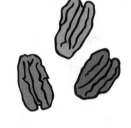

MAKES 9 BLONDIES
MILK MAKER: oats
SUPERFOODS: chickpeas, almond butter, pecans

1½ cups (250 g) cooked chickpeas
½ cup (125 g) almond butter
⅓ cup (65 g) sugar
¼ cup (60 ml) maple syrup
¼ cup (20 g) rolled oats
1 teaspoon ground cinnamon

1 teaspoon vanilla extract
½ teaspoon baking powder
½ teaspoon ground cardamom
¼ teaspoon baking soda
¼ teaspoon salt
¼ cup (25 g) chopped pecans

1. Preheat the oven to 350°F (180°C). Line an 8-inch (20 cm) square baking dish with parchment paper.

2. Process all the ingredients except the pecans in a food processor until smooth. Add the pecans and pulse three times to incorporate into the batter. Transfer to the prepared baking dish.

3. Bake for 25 to 30 minutes, until the blondies begin to firm up at the top and pull away from the sides of the parchment paper. Remove from the oven and allow to cool completely before cutting into nine squares and serving.

PER BLONDIE Calories: 210; total fat: 11 g; saturated fat: 1 g; cholesterol: 0 mg/dl; sodium: 105 mg; total carbohydrate: 26 g; dietary fiber: 4 g; sugar: 16 g; protein: 6 g; vitamin A: 0 mcg; vitamin C: 0 mg; calcium: 78 mg; iron: 1.4 mg

Rich in vitamin E, riboflavin, folate, phosphorus, magnesium, zinc, copper, and manganese

Classic Sugar Cookies

MAKES 24 COOKIES
SUPERFOODS: chia seeds, almonds

½ cup (120 ml) water

2 tablespoons ground chia seeds

¾ cup (150 g) sugar

¾ cup (170 g) Earth Balance margarine, softened

1 teaspoon vanilla extract

½ teaspoon baking soda

¼ teaspoon salt

2¼ cups (250 g) almond flour, plus more for dusting

½ cup (60 g) coconut flour

1. Whisk the water and chia seeds together in a small bowl until combined; set aside.

2. Using an electric mixer, cream the sugar and margarine in a large bowl. Add the vanilla, baking soda, salt, and chia seed mixture; mix for an additional 30 seconds. Add the almond flour and beat until combined. Add the coconut flour and mix until a soft dough starts to form.

3. Form the dough into a large ball, wrap in plastic wrap, and refrigerate for at least 30 minutes or overnight.

4. Preheat the oven to 350°F (180°C). Line one large or two medium baking sheets with parchment paper.

RECIPE CONTINUES →

5. Lightly flour a clean, flat surface with almond flour. Roll out the dough to ¼ inch (6 mm) thick and, using your choice of cookie cutters, cut out cookies and place on the prepared baking sheet about 2 inches (5 cm) apart. Continue rolling and cutting until all the dough is used. If you're in a rush, use a pizza cutter or knife to cut the dough into triangles, rectangles, or squares and place on the baking sheet.

6. For soft and chewy cookies, bake for about 13 minutes, and for crispier cookies, bake for about 15 minutes. These cookies go from soft and chewy to crispy in just a matter of minutes, so be sure to set a timer and watch them closely. They will appear soft no matter when you take them out of the oven, but they will harden as they cool. Transfer the cookies to a wire rack and allow to cool to room temperature before enjoying. The cookies will keep for 3 to 5 days in an airtight container and also freeze well.

PER COOKIE Calories: 150; total fat: 11 g; saturated fat: 2 g; cholesterol: 0 mg/dl; sodium: 110 mg; total carbohydrate: 10 g; dietary fiber: 2 g; sugar: 7 g; protein: 3 g; vitamin A: 0 mcg; vitamin C: 0 mg; calcium: 26 mg; iron: 0.4 mg
Rich in vitamin E

Avocado Ice Cream

MAKES 1 QUART (1 L)
SUPERFOODS: avocado, kale

2 Hass avocados, halved and pitted
One 13.5-ounce (400 ml) can coconut milk
½ cup (125 g) frozen kale
½ cup (100 g) raw/turbinado sugar
1 tablespoon fresh lime or lemon juice
1 tablespoon powdered calcium citrate, optional

1. Scoop the avocado flesh into a blender or food processor. Add the remaining ingredients and blend until smooth.

2. Transfer to an ice cream maker and process according to the manufacturer's directions.

3. Transfer to a 1-quart (1 L) freezer-safe container and freeze for an additional 2 hours to firm to a delightful ice cream texture.

PER SERVING (¼ CUP/60 ML; 8 SERVINGS PER RECIPE), NOT INCLUDING CALCIUM CITRATE Calories: 210; total fat: 16 g; saturated fat: 10 g; cholesterol: 0 mg/dl; sodium: 10 mg; total carbohydrate: 18 g; dietary fiber: 3 g; sugar: 13 g; protein: 2 g; vitamin A: 600 mcg; vitamin C: 9 mg; calcium: 0 mg; iron: 1.8 mg

Rich in iron, vitamin A, vitamin C, folate, pantothenic acid, copper, and manganese

PER SERVING (¼ CUP/60 ML; 8 SERVINGS PER RECIPE), INCLUDING CALCIUM CITRATE Calories: 210; total fat: 16 g; saturated fat: 10 g; cholesterol: 0 mg/dl; sodium: 10 mg; total carbohydrate: 18 g; dietary fiber: 3 g; sugar: 13 g; protein: 2 g; vitamin A: 600 mcg; vitamin C: 9 mg; calcium: 195 mg; iron: 1.8 mg

Rich in calcium, iron, vitamin A, vitamin C, folate, pantothenic acid, copper, and manganese

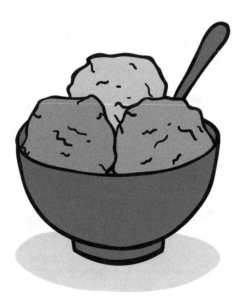

NOTES

CHAPTER 2

1. Blyth, R., et al., "Effect of Maternal Confidence on Breastfeeding Duration: An Application of Breastfeeding Self-Efficacy Theory," *Birth* 29, no. 4 (2002): 278–84.

    Brand, E., C. Kothari, and M. A. Stark, "Factors Related to Breastfeeding Discontinuation Between Hospital Discharge and 2 Weeks Postpartum," *Journal of Perinatal Education* 20, no. 1 (2011): 36–44.

    Chezem, J., C. Friesen, and J. Boettcher, "Breastfeeding Knowledge, Breastfeeding Confidence, and Infant Feeding Plans: Effects on Actual Feeding Practices," *Journal of Obstetric, Gynecologic, and Neonatal Nursing* 32, no. 1 (2003): 40–47.

    Dennis, C. L., "Theoretical Underpinings of Breastfeeding Confidence: A Self-Efficacy Framework," *Journal of Human Lactation* 15, no. 3 (1999): 195–201.

    Grassley, J. S., and T. P. Nelms, "Understanding Maternal Breastfeeding Confidence: A Gadamerian Hermeneutic Analysis of Women's Stories," *Health Care for Women International* 29, no. 8 (2008): 841–62.

    Jones, J. R., et al., "Factors Associated with Exclusive Breastfeeding in the United States," *Pediatrics* 128, no. 6 (2011): 1117–25.

    McCarter-Spaulding, D., and R. Gore, "Breastfeeding Self-Efficacy in Women of African Descent," *Journal of Obstetric, Gynecologic, and Neonatal Nursing* 38, no. 2 (2009): 230–43.

    Mossman, M., et al., "The Influence of Adolescent Mothers' Breastfeeding Confidence and Attitudes on Breastfeeding Initiation and Duration," *Journal of Human Lactation* 24, no. 3 (2008): p. 268–77.

    Nommsen-Rivers, L. A., and K. G. Dewey, "Development and Validation of the Infant Feeding Intentions Scale," *Maternal and Child Health Journal* 13, no. 3 (2009): 334–42.

    Robinson, K. M., "African American Women's Infant Feeding Choices: Analyzing Self-Efficacy and Narratives from a Black Feminist Perspective" (dissertation, Marquette University, 2010), 187.

    Larsen, J. S., E. O. Hall, and H. Aagaard, "Shattered Expectations: When Mothers' Confidence in Breastfeeding Is Undermined—A Metasynthesis," *Scandinavian Journal of Caring Sciences* 22, no. 4 (2008): 653–61.

    Simpson, A. C., "Sociocultural Barriers to Breast Feeding in African American Women with Focused Intervention to Increased Prevalence" (master's thesis, Georgia State University, 2012).

CHAPTER 3

1. Liu, X., et al., "Stat5a Is Mandatory for Adult Mammary Gland Development and Lactogenesis," *Genes and Development* 11, no. 2 (1997): 179–86.

2. Neville, M. C., and J. Morton, "Physiology and Endocrine Changes Underlying Human Lactogenesis II," *Journal of Nutrition* 131, no. 11: 3005S–8S.

3. Godhia, M. L., and N. Patel, "Colostrum–Its Composition, Benefits as a Nutraceutical–A Review," *Current Research in Nutrition and Food Science* 1, no. 1 (2013): 37–47.
   Hurley, W. L., and P. K. Theil, "Perspectives on Immunoglobulins in Colostrum and Milk," *Nutrients* 3, no. 4 (2011): 442–74.

4. Hill, P. D., R. T. Chatterton, and J. C. Aldag Jr., "Serum Prolactin in Breastfeeding: State of the Science," *Biological Research for Nursing* 1, no. 1 (1999): 65–75.

5. Ibid.

6. Vallone, S., "Role of Subluxation and Chiropractic Care in Hypolactation," *Journal of Clinical Chiropractic Pediatrics* 8, nos. 1 and 2 (2007): 518–24.

7. Gimpl, G., and F. Fahrenholz, "The Oxytocin Receptor System: Structure, Function, and Regulation," *Physiological Reviews* 81, no. 2 (2001): 629–83.
   Guastella, A. J., P. B. Mitchell, and M. R. Dadds, "Oxytocin Increases Gaze to the Eye Region of Human Faces," *Biological Psychiatry* 63, no. 1 (2008): 3–5.
   Kirsch, P., et al., "Oxytocin Modulates Neural Circuitry for Social Cognition and Fear in Humans," *Journal of Neuroscience* 25, no. 49 (2005): 11489–93.
   Kosfeld, M., et al., "Oxytocin Increases Trust in Humans," *Nature* 435, no. 7042 (2005): 673–76.
   Moberg, K. U., *The Oxytocin Factor: Tapping the Hormone of Calm, Love, and Healing* (Cambridge, MA: Da Capo Press, 2003).

8. Donaldson-Myles, F., "Can Hormones in Breastfeeding Protect Against Postnatal Depression?" *British Journal of Midwifery* 20, no. 2 (2012): 88–93.

9. Zanardo, V., et al., "Impaired Lactation Performance Following Elective Delivery at Term: Role of Maternal Levels of Cortisol and Prolactin," *Journal of Maternal-Fetal and Neonatal Medicine* 25, no. 9 (2012): 1595–98.

10. Ibid.

CHAPTER 4

1. Garber, M., "A Brief History of Breast Pumps," *Atlantic*, October 21, 2013.

2. Academy of Breastfeeding Medicine Protocol Committee, "ABM Clinical Protocol #3: Hospital Guidelines for the Use of Supplementary Feedings in the Healthy Term Breastfed Neonate, Revised 2009," *Breastfeeding Medicine* 4, no. 3 (2009).

3. Flaherman, V. J., et al., "Early Weight Loss Nomograms for Exclusively Breastfed Newborns," *Pediatrics* 135, no. 1 (2015): e16–e23.

4. Hirth, R., T. Weitkamp, and A. Dwivedi, "Maternal Intravenous Fluids and Infant Weight," *Clinical Lactation* 3, no. 2 (2012): p. 59–63.

5. Miller, J. R., et al., "Early Weight Loss Nomograms for Formula Fed Newborns," *Hospital Pediatrics* 5, no. 5 (2015): 263–68.

CHAPTER 5

1. Marshall, D. R., P. P. Callan, and W. Nicholson, "Breastfeeding After Reduction Mammaplasty," *British Journal of Plastic Surgery* 47, no. 3 (1994): 167–69.
   Souto, G. C., et al., "The Impact of Breast Reduction Surgery on Breastfeeding Performance," *Journal of Human Lactation* 19, no. 1 (2003): 43–49.

2. Betzold, C. M., "An Update on the Recognition and Management of Lactational Breast Inflammation," *Journal of Midwifery and Women's Health* 52, no. 6 (2007): 595–605.
3. World Health Organization, *Mastitis: Causes and Management* (Geneva: World Health Organization, 2000).
4. Ibid.
5. Academy of Breastfeeding Medicine Protocol Committee, "ABM Clinical Protocol #4: Mastitis, Revised March 2014," *Breastfeeding Medicine* 9, no. 5 (2014).
6. Fetherston, C., "Risk Factors for Lactation Mastitis," *Journal of Human Lactation* 14, no. 2 (1998): 101–9.

    Foxman, B., et al., "Lactation Mastitis: Occurrence and Medical Management Among 946 Breastfeeding Women in the United States," *American Journal of Epidemiology* 155, no. 2 (2002): 103–14.

    Kinlay, J. R., D. L. O'Connell, and S. Kinlay, "Risk Factors for Mastitis in Breastfeeding Women: Results of a Prospective Cohort Study," *Australian and New Zealand Journal of Public Health* 25, no. 2 (2001): 115–20.
7. Neifert, M. R., J. M. Seacat, and W. E. Jobe, "Lactation Failure Due to Insufficient Glandular Development of the Breast," *Pediatrics* 76, no. 5 (1985): 823–28.
8. Britz, S. P., and L. Henry, "PCOS and Breastfeeding: What's the Issue?" *Journal of Obstetric, Gynecologic, and Neonatal Nursing* 40 (2011): S127.

    Vanky, E., et al., "Breastfeeding in Polycystic Ovary Syndrome," *Acta Obstetricia et Gynecologica Scandinavica* 87, no. 5 (2008): 531–35.
9. Mayo Clinic Staff, "Diseases and Conditions: Polycystic Ovary Syndrome (PCOS)," mayoclinic.org, September 3, 2014.
10. Carlsen, S., G. Jacobsen, and E. Vanky, "Mid-Pregnancy Androgen Levels Are Negatively Associated with Breastfeeding," *Acta Obstetricia et Gynecologica Scandinavica* 89, no. 1 (2010): 87–94.
11. Speller, E., W. Brodribb, and E. McGuire, "Breastfeeding and Thyroid Disease: A Literature Review," *Breastfeeding Review* 20, no. 2 (2012): 41.
12. Amino, N., et al., "Transient Postpartum Hypothyroidism: Fourteen Cases with Autoimmune Thyroiditis," *Annals of Internal Medicine* 87, no. 2 (1977): 155–59.
13. Riordan, J., and K. Wambach, *Breastfeeding and Human Lactation*, 4th ed. (Burlington, MA: Jones & Bartlett Learning, 2009).
14. Hill, Chatterton, and Aldag, "Serum Prolactin in Breastfeeding: State of the Science."
15. Baser, H., et al., "The Incidence of Postpartum Thyroiditis at First Month Postpartum," *Pakistan Journal of Medical Sciences* 27, no. 5 (2011): 1079–82.
16. Groer, M., and C. Jevitt, "Symptoms and Signs Associated with Postpartum Thyroiditis," *Journal of Thyroid Research* 2014 (2014): 1–6.
17. Baser et al., "The Incidence of Postpartum Thyroiditis at First Month Postpartum."
18. Groer and Jevitt, "Symptoms and Signs Associated with Postpartum Thyroiditis."
19. Benson, C. T., and G. T. Griffing, "Prolactin Deficiency," medscape.com, June 10, 2014.
20. Bachelot, A., and N. Binart, "Reproductive Role of Prolactin," *Reproduction* 133, no. 2 (2007): 361–69.
21. Ozkan, Y., and R. Colak, "Sheehan Syndrome: Clinical and Laboratory Evaluation of 20 Cases," *Neuroendocrinology Letters* 26, no. 3 (2005): 257–60.
22. Labbok, M. H., et al., "Multicenter Study of the Lactational Amenorrhea Method (LAM): I. Efficacy, Duration, and Implications for Clinical Application," *Contraception* 55, no. 6 (1997): 327–36.

Kennedy, K. I., M. H. Labbok, and P. F. A. Van Look, "Lactational Amenorrhea Method for Family Planning," *International Journal of Gynecology and Obstetrics* 54, no. 1 (1996): 55–57.

23. Phillips, S. J., et al., "Progestogen-Only Contraceptive Use Among Breastfeeding Women: A Systematic Review," *Contraception* 94, no. 3 (2016): 226–52.

24. Ibid.; Brownell, E. A., et al., "The Effect of Immediate Postpartum Depot Medroxyprogesterone on Early Breastfeeding Cessation," *Contraception* 87, no. 6 (2013): 836–43.

25. Braga, G. C., et al., "Immediate Postpartum Initiation of Etonogestrel-Releasing Implant: A Randomized Controlled Trial on Breastfeeding Impact," *Contraception* 92, no. 6 (2015): 536–42.

26. Tepper, N. K., et al., "Combined Hormonal Contraceptive Use Among Breastfeeding Women: An Updated Systematic Review," *Contraception* 94, no. 3 (2016): 262–74.

27. Toddywalla, V. S., et al., "Is Time-Interval Between Mini-Pill Ingestion and Breastfeeding Essential?" *Contraception* 51, no. 3 (1995): 193–95.

28. Kotlow, L. A., "Ankyloglossia (Tongue-Tie): A Diagnostic and Treatment Quandary," *Quintessence International* 30, no. 4 (1999): p. 259–62.

Pransky, S. M., D. Lago, and P. Hong, "Breastfeeding Difficulties and Oral Cavity Anomalies: The Influence of Posterior Ankyloglossia and Upper-Lip Ties," *International Journal of Pediatric Otorhinolaryngology* 79, no. 10 (2015): 1714–17.

Rowan-Legg, A., "Ankyloglossia and Breastfeeding," *Paediatrics and Child Health* 16, no. 4 (2011): 222.

29. Macaluso, M., and D. Hockenbury, "Lingual and Labial Frenums: Early Detection Can Prevent Cascading Health Effects Associated with Tongue-Tie," *RDH* 35, no. 12 (2015): 48–51.

30. Ibid.

31. Ibid.; Rowan-Legg, "Ankyloglossia and Breastfeeding."

32. Pransky, Lago, and Hong, "Breastfeeding Difficulties and Oral Cavity Anomalies."

33. Ibid.; Ito, Y., "Does Frenotomy Improve Breast-Feeding Difficulties in Infants with Ankyloglossia?" *Pediatrics International* 56, no. 4 (2014): 497–505.

34. Ibid.

35. Fry, L. M., "Chiropractic and Breastfeeding Dysfunction: A Literature Review," *Journal of Clinical Chiropractic Pediatrics* 14, no. 2 (2014): 1151–55.

36. Garcez, L. W., and E. R. Giugliani, "Population-Based Study on the Practice of Breastfeeding in Children Born with Cleft Lip and Palate," *Cleft Palate-Craniofacial Journal* 42, no. 6 (2005): 687–93.

37. Zanardo et al., "Impaired Lactation Performance Following Elective Delivery at Term."

38. Noel-Weiss, J., et al., "An Observational Study of Associations Among Maternal Fluids During Parturition, Neonatal Output, and Breastfed Newborn Weight Loss," *International Breastfeeding Journal* 6, no. 9 (2011).

39. Zanardo et al., "Impaired Lactation Performance Following Elective Delivery at Term."

40. Neville and Morton, "Physiology and Endocrine Changes Underlying Human Lactogenesis II."

41. Rasmussen, K. M., and C. L. Kjolhede, "Prepregnant Overweight and Obesity Diminish the Prolactin Response to Suckling in the First Week Postpartum," *Pediatrics* 113, no. 5 (2004): e465–71.

42. Ibid.

43. Rasmussen, K. M., J. A. Hilson, and C. L. Kjolhede, "Obesity May Impair Lactogenesis II," *Journal of Nutrition* 131, no. 11 (2001): 3009S–11S

Nommsen-Rivers, L. A., et al., "Delayed Onset of Lactogenesis Among First-Time Mothers Is Related to Maternal Obesity and Factors Associated with Ineffective Breastfeeding," *American Journal of Clinical Nutrition* 92, no. 3 (2010): 574–84.

CHAPTER 6

1. Chertok, I. R., "Reexamination of Ultra-Thin Nipple Shield Use, Infant Growth and Maternal Satisfaction," *Journal of Clinical Nursing* 18, no. 21 (2009): 2949–55.

Brigham, M., "Mothers' Reports of the Outcome of Nipple Shield Use," *Journal of Human Lactation* 12, no. 4 (1996): 291–97.

2. Amir, L. H., "Breast Pain in Lactating Women—Mastitis or Something Else?" *Australian Family Physician* 32, no. 3 (2003): 141.

Berens, P. D., "Breast Pain: Engorgement, Nipple Pain and Mastitis," *Clinical Obstetrics and Gynecology* 58, no. 4 (2015): 902–14.

3. Academy of Breastfeeding Medicine Protocol Committee, "ABM Clinical Protocol #3."

4. Ibid.

5. Wright, C., and K. Parkinson, "Postnatal Weight Loss in Term Infants: What Is 'Normal' and Do Growth Charts Allow for It?" *Archives of Disease in Childhood–Fetal and Neonatal Edition* 89, no. 3 (2004): F254–57.

6. Martens, P. J., and L. Romphf, "Factors Associated with Newborn In-Hospital Weight Loss: Comparisons by Feeding Method, Demographics, and Birthing Procedures," *Journal of Human Lactation* 23, no. 3 (2007): 233–41.

7. Noel-Weiss et al., "An Observational Study of Associations Among Maternal Fluids During Parturition, Neonatal Output, and Breastfed Newborn Weight Loss."

8. Cabar, H. D., A. Aydin, and U. Gullu, "Care in Neonatal Jaundice," *International Journal of Academic Research* 6, no. 3 (2014): 8–14.

9. Academy of Breastfeeding Medicine Protocol Committee, "ABM Clinical Protocol #3."

10. Cabar, Aydin, and Gullu, "Care in Neonatal Jaundice."

11. Academy of Breastfeeding Medicine Protocol Committee, "ABM Clinical Protocol #3."

12. Academy of Breastfeeding Medicine Protocol Committee, "ABM Clinical Protocol #22: Guidelines for Management of Jaundice in the Breastfeeding Infant Equal to or Greater than 35 Weeks' Gestation," *Breastfeeding Medicine* 5, no. 2 (2010): 87.

Soldi, A., et al., "Neonatal Jaundice and Human Milk," *Journal of Maternal-Fetal and Neonatal Medicine* 24, no. S1 (2011): 85–87.

13. Academy of Breastfeeding Medicine Protocol Committee, "ABM Clinical Protocol #22."

14. Hill, Chatterton, and Aldag, "Serum Prolactin in Breastfeeding: State of the Science."

15. Aney, M., "'Babywise' Advice Linked to Dehydration, Failure to Thrive," *AAP News* 14, no. 4 (1998): 21.

16. Galland, B. C., et al., "Normal Sleep Patterns in Infants and Children: A Systematic Review of Observational Studies," *Sleep Medicine Reviews* 16, no. 3 (2012): 213–22.

17. Delgado, H. L., A. S. McNeilly, and P. E. Hartmann, "Non-Nutritional Factors Affecting Milk Production," in *Maternal Diet, Breast-Feeding Capacity, and Lactational Infertility*, ed. R. G. Whitehead (Tokyo: United Nations University Press, 1983), 54–62.

18. Bronner, Y. L., et al., "Early Introduction of Solid Foods Among Urban African-American Participants in WIC," *Journal of the American Dietetic Association* 99, no. 4 (1999): 457–61.

19. Ibid.; Scott, J. A., et al., "Predictors of the Early Introduction of Solid Foods in Infants: Results of a Cohort Study," *BMC Pediatrics* 9, no. 1 (2009): 60.

20. Crocetti, M., R. Dudas, and S. Krugman, "Parental Beliefs and Practices Regarding Early Introduction of Solid Foods to Their Children," *Clinical Pediatrics* 43, no. 6 (2004): 541–47.

21. Delgado, McNeilly, and Hartmann, "Non-Nutritional Factors Affecting Milk Production."

CHAPTER 7

1. Whitehead, R. G., ed., *Maternal Diet, Breast-Feeding Capacity, and Lactational Infertility* (Tokyo: The United Nations University Press, 1983).

2. Ibid.

3. Jadhav, A. N., and K. K. Bhutani, "Ayurveda and Gynecological Disorders," *Journal of Ethnopharmacology* 91, no. 1 (2005): 151–59.

   Buhrman, S., "Ayurvedic Approaches to Women's Health," *Protocol Journal of Botanic Medicine* 1, no. 4 (1996): 2–7.

4. Hill, Chatterton, and Aldag, "Serum Prolactin in Breastfeeding: State of the Science."

CHAPTER 8

1. Saarinen, U. M., and M. Kajosaari, "Breastfeeding as Prophylaxis Against Atopic Disease: Prospective Follow-Up Study Until 17 Years Old," *Lancet* 346, no. 8982 (1995): 1065–69.

   van Odijk, J., et al., "Breastfeeding and Allergic Disease: A Multidisciplinary Review of the Literature (1966–2001) on the Mode of Early Feeding in Infancy and Its Impact on Later Atopic Manifestations," *Allergy* 58, no. 9 (2003): 833–43.

2. Greer, F. R., et al., "Effects of Early Nutritional Interventions on the Development of Atopic Disease in Infants and Children: The Role of Maternal Dietary Restriction, Breastfeeding, Timing of Introduction of Complementary Foods, and Hydrolyzed Formulas," *Pediatrics* 121, no. 1 (2008): 183–91.

3. Norman, J. E., and R. M. Reynolds, "The Consequences of Obesity and Excess Weight Gain in Pregnancy," *Proceedings of the Nutrition Society* 70, no. 4 (2011): 450–56.

4. Mamun, A. A., et al., "Associations of Maternal Pre-Pregnancy Obesity and Excess Pregnancy Weight Gains with Adverse Pregnancy Outcomes and Length of Hospital Stay," *BMC Pregnancy and Childbirth* 11, no. 1 (2011): 62.

   Ekblad, U., and S. Grenman, "Maternal Weight, Weight Gain During Pregnancy and Pregnancy Outcome," *International Journal of Gynaecology and Obstetrics* 39, no. 4 (1992): 277–83.

5. Norman and Reynolds, "The Consequences of Obesity and Excess Weight Gain in Pregnancy."

   Crane, J., et al., "The Effect of Gestational Weight Gain by Body Mass Index on Maternal and Neonatal Outcomes," *Journal of Obstetrics and Gynaecology Canada* 31, no. 1 (2009): 28–35.

   Chu, S. Y., et al., "Maternal Obesity and Risk of Stillbirth: A Metaanalysis," *American Journal of Obstetrics and Gynecology* 197, no. 3 (2007): 223–28.

   Olafsdottir, A., et al., "Maternal Diet in Early and Late Pregnancy in Relation to Weight Gain," *International Journal of Obesity* 30, no. 3 (2006): 492–99.

6. Siega-Riz, A. M., L. S. Adair, and C. J. Hobel, "Maternal Underweight Status and Inadequate Rate of Weight Gain During the Third Trimester of Pregnancy Increases the Risk of Preterm Delivery," *Journal of Nutrition* 126, no. 1 (1996): 146–53.

7. K. M. Rasmussen and A. L. Yaktine, eds., *Weight Gain During Pregnancy: Reexamining the Guidelines*, Institute of Medicine Report Brief (Washington, DC: National Academies Press, 2009).

Polley, B. A., R. Wing, and C. Sims, "Randomized Controlled Trial to Prevent Excessive Weight Gain in Pregnant Women," *International Journal of Obesity and Related Metabolic Disorders* 26, no. 11 (2002): 1494–1502.

Artal, R., C. J. Lockwood, and H. L. Brown, "Weight Gain Recommendations in Pregnancy and the Obesity Epidemic," *Obstetrics and Gynecology* 115, no. 1 (2010): 152–55.

8. Polley, Wing, and Sims, "Randomized Controlled Trial to Prevent Excessive Weight Gain in Pregnant Women."

Keppel, K. G., and S. M. Taffel, "Pregnancy-Related Weight Gain and Retention: Implications of the 1990 Institute of Medicine Guidelines," *American Journal of Public Health* 83, no. 8 (1993): 1100–1103.

Gunderson, E. P., and B. Abrams, "Epidemiology of Gestational Weight Gain and Body Weight Changes After Pregnancy," *Epidemiologic Reviews* 22, no. 2 (1999): 261–74.

Ohlin, A., and S. Rössner, "Maternal Body Weight Development After Pregnancy," *International Journal of Obesity* 14, no. 2 (1990): 159–73.

Schauberger, C. W., B. L. Rooney, and L. M. Brimer, "Factors That Influence Weight Loss in the Puerperium," *Obstetrics and Gynecology* 79, no. 3 (1992): 424–29.

9. Dewey, K. G., M. J. Heinig, and L. A. Nommsen, "Maternal Weight-Loss Patterns During Prolonged Lactation," *American Journal of Clinical Nutrition* 58, no. 2 (1993): 162–66.

Dewey, K. G., "Impact of Breastfeeding on Maternal Nutritional Status," in *Protecting Infants Through Human Milk*, ed. L. K. Pickering et al. (New York: Springer, 2004), 91–100.

Dewey, K. G., et al., "Effects of Exclusive Breastfeeding for Four Versus Six Months on Maternal Nutritional Status and Infant Motor Development: Results of Two Randomized Trials in Honduras," *Journal of Nutrition* 131, no. 2 (2001): 262–67.

10. Lovelady, C. A., et al., "The Effect of Weight Loss in Overweight, Lactating Women on the Growth of Their Infants," *New England Journal of Medicine* 342, no. 7 (2000): 449–53.

Dewey, K. G., "Effects of Maternal Caloric Restriction and Exercise During Lactation," *Journal of Nutrition* 128, no. 2 (1998): 386S–89S.

McCrory, M. A., et al., "Randomized Trial of the Short-Term Effects of Dieting Compared with Dieting Plus Aerobic Exercise on Lactation Performance," *American Journal of Clinical Nutrition* 69, no 5 (1999): 959–67.

11. McCrory et al., "Randomized Trial of the Short-Term Effects of Dieting Compared with Dieting Plus Aerobic Exercise on Lactation Performance."

12. Ibid.; Dewey, "Effects of Maternal Caloric Restriction and Exercise During Lactation."

13. Dewey, Heinig, and Nommsen, "Maternal Weight-Loss Patterns During Prolonged Lactation."

14. Innis, S. M., "Dietary Omega 3 Fatty Acids and the Developing Brain," *Brain Research* 1237 (2008): 35–43.

15. Bernard, J. Y., et al., "The Dietary n6:n3 Fatty Acid Ratio During Pregnancy Is Inversely Associated with Child Neurodevelopment in the EDEN Mother-Child Cohort," *Journal of Nutrition* 143, no. 9 (2013): 1481–88.

16. Antonakou, A., et al., "Breast Milk Fat Concentration and Fatty Acid Pattern During the First Six Months in Exclusively Breastfeeding Greek Women," *European Journal of Nutrition* 52, no. 3 (2013): 963–73.

17. Allen, N. E., et al., "Animal Foods, Protein, Calcium and Prostate Cancer Risk: The European Prospective Investigation into Cancer and Nutrition," *British Journal of Cancer* 98, no. 9 (2008): 1574–81.

Fulgoni, V. L., III, "Current Protein Intake in America: Analysis of the National Health and Nutrition Examination Survey, 2003–2004," *American Journal of Clinical Nutrition* 87, no. 5 (2008): 1554S–57S.

Lowery, L. M., and L. Devia, "Dietary Protein Safety and Resistance Exercise: What Do We Really Know?" *Journal of the International Society of Sports Nutrition* 6, no. 3 (2009): 1.

Food and Agriculture Organization of the United Nations, Statistics Division, 2010.

de Boer, J., M. Helms, and H. Aiking, "Protein Consumption and Sustainability: Diet Diversity in EU-15," *Ecological Economics* 59, no. 3 (2006): 267–74.

Feskanich, D., et al., "Protein Consumption and Bone Fractures in Women," *American Journal of Epidemiology* 143, no. 5 (1996): 472–79.

Metges, C. C., and C. A. Barth, "Metabolic Consequences of a High Dietary-Protein Intake in Adulthood: Assessment of the Available Evidence," *Journal of Nutrition* 130, no. 4 (2000): 886–89.

Brändle, E., H. G. Sieberth, and R. E. Hautmann, "Effect of Chronic Dietary Protein Intake on the Renal Function in Healthy Subjects," *European Journal of Clinical Nutrition* 50, no. 11 (1996): 734–40.

CHAPTER 9

1. Koletzko, B., and F. Lehner, "Beer and Breastfeeding," in *Short and Long Term Effects of Breast Feeding on Child Health*, ed. B. Koletzko, K. Fleischer Michaelsen, and O. Hernell (New York: Springer, 2002), 23–28.

Sawadogo, L., and L. M. Houdebine, "Identification of the Lactogenic Compound Present in Beer," *Annales de biologie clinique* 46, no. 2 (1988): 129–34.

2. Sawadogo, L., H. Sepehri, and L. M. Houdebine, "Evidence for Stimulating Factor of Prolactin and Growth Hormone Secretion Present in Brewery Draff," *Reproduction, Nutrition, Development* 29, no. 2 (1989): 139–46.

3. Sawadogo and Houdebine, "Identification of the Lactogenic Compound Present in Beer."

4. Webb, D., "Betting on Beta-Glucans," *Today's Dietitian* 16, no. 5 (2014): 16.

5. Sambou Diatta, B. "Supplementation for Pregnant and Breastfeeding Women with *Moringa oleifera* Powder," paper presented at Development Potential for Moringa Products, international workshop, Dar es Salaam, Tanzania, October 29–November 2, 2001.

6. Dhakar, R. C., et al., "Moringa: The Herbal Gold to Combat Malnutrition," *Chronicles of Young Scientists* 2, no. 3 (2011): 119.

7. Nweze, N. O., and F. I. Nwafor, "Phytochemical, Proximate and Mineral Composition of Leaf Extracts of *Moringa oleifera* Lam. from Nsukka, South-Eastern Nigeria," *IOSR Journal of Pharmacy and Biological Sciences* 9, no. 1 (2014): 99–103.

8. Dhakar et al., "Moringa: The Herbal Gold to Combat Malnutrition."

9. Raguindin, P., L. F. Dans, and J. F. King, "*Moringa oleifera* as a Galactagogue," *Breastfeeding Medicine* 9, no. 6 (2014): 323–24.

10. Yabes-Almirante, C., and M. Lim, "Effectiveness of Natalac as a Galactogogue," *Journal of Philippine Medical Association* 71, no. 3 (1996): 265–72.

11. Raguindin, Dans, and King, "*Moringa oleifera* as a Galactagogue."

12. Estrella, M. C. P., et al., "A Double-Blind, Randomized Controlled Trial on the Use of Malunggay (*Moringa oleifera*) for Augmentation of the Volume of Breastmilk Among Non-Nursing Mothers of Preterm Infants," *Philippine Journal of Pediatrics* 49, no. 1 (2000): 3.

13. Balahibo, M. F., et al., "A Randomized, Double-Blinded Parralel-Controlled Clinical Trial on the Effectiveness of Different Doses of *Moringa oleifera* (Malunggay) in Promoting Growth in Infants of Breastfeeding Mothers from the UERMMMC and Different Hospitals in Metro Manila from June 2000 to January 2001," *UERMMMC Journal of Health Sciences* 5, no. 1 (2002): 21–26.

14. Estrella et al., "A Double-Blind, Randomized Controlled Trial on the Use of Malunggay (*Moringa oleifera*) for Augmentation of the Volume of Breastmilk Among Non-Nursing Mothers of Preterm Infants."

    Balahibo et al., "A Randomized, Double-Blinded Parralel-Controlled Clinical Trial on the Effectiveness of Different Doses of *Moringa oleifera* (Malunggay) in Promoting Growth in Infants of Breastfeeding Mothers from the UERMMMC and Different Hospitals in Metro Manila from June 2000 to January 2001."

    Epsinosa-Kuo, C. L., "A Randomized Controlled Trial on the Use of Malunggay (*Moringa oleifera*) for Augmentation of the Volume of Breastmilk Among Mothers of Term Infants," *Filipino Family Physician* 43, no. 1 (2005): 26–33.

15. Epsinosa-Kuo, "A Randomized Controlled Trial on the Use of Malunggay (*Moringa oleifera*) for Augmentation of the Volume of Breastmilk Among Mothers of Term Infants."

16. Shen, Y. B., et al., "Effects of Supplementing Saccharomyces Cerevisiae Fermentation Product in Sow Diets on Performance of Sows and Nursing Piglets," *Journal of Animal Science* 89, no. 8 (2011): 2462–71.

    LeMieux, F. M., et al., "Effect of Dried Brewers Yeast on Growth Performance of Nursing and Weanling Pigs," *Professional Animal Scientist* 26, no. 1 (2010): 70–75.

17. Shen et al., "Effects of Supplementing Saccharomyces Cerevisiae Fermentation Product in Sow Diets on Performance of Sows and Nursing Piglets."

18. Smith, M., et al., "Therapeutic Applications of Fenugreek," *Alternative Medicine Review* 8, no. 1 (2003): 20–27.

19. El Sakka, A., M. Salama, and K. Salama, "The Effect of Fenugreek Herbal Tea and Palm Dates on Breast Milk Production and Infant Weight," *Journal of Pediatric Sciences* 6 (2014).

20. Forinash, A. B., et al., "The Use of Galactogogues in the Breastfeeding Mother," *Annals of Pharmacotherapy* 46, no. 10 (2012): 1392–404.

    Zapantis, A., J. G. Steinberg, and L. Schilit, "Use of Herbal Galactagogues," *Journal of Pharmacy Practice* 25, no. 2 (2012): 222–31.

21. Huggins, K. E., "Fenugreek: One Remedy for Low Milk Production," breastfeedingonline. com, 2012.

22. Smith et al., "Therapeutic Applications of Fenugreek."

23. Academy of Breastfeeding Medicine Protocol Committee, "ABM Clinical Protocol# 9: Use of Galactogogues in Initiating or Augmenting the Rate of Maternal Milk Secretion (First Revision January 2011)," *Breastfeeding Medicine* 6, no. 1 (2011): 41–49.

24. Gufford, B. T., et al., "Chemoenzymatic Synthesis, Characterization, and Scale-Up of Milk Thistle Flavonolignan Glucuronides," *Drug Metabolism and Disposition* 43, no. 11 (2015): 1734–43.

25. Academy of Breastfeeding Medicine Protocol Committee, "ABM Clinical Protocol# 9."
26. Gufford, B. T., et al., "Milk Thistle Constituents Inhibit Raloxifene Intestinal Glucuronidation: A Potential Clinically Relevant Natural Product-Drug Interaction," *Drug Metabolism and Disposition* 43, no. 9 (2015): 1353–59.
27. Gupta, M., and B. Shaw, "A Double-Blind Randomized Clinical Trial for Evaluation of Galactogogue Acticity of *Asparagus racemosus* Willd," *Iranian Journal of Pharmaceutical Research* 10, no. 1 (2011): 167–72.
28. Ibid.; Sayed, N. Z., R. Deo, and U. Mukundan, "Herbal Remedies Used by Warlis of Dahanu to Induce Lactation in Nursing Mothers," *Indian Journal of Traditional Knowledge* 6, no. 4 (2007): 602–5.
29. Jadhav, A. N., and K. Bhutani, "Ayurveda and Gynecological Disorders," Journal of *Ethnopharmacology* 97, no. 1 (2005): 151–59.
    Buhrman, S., "Ayurvedic Approaches to Women's Health," *Protocol Journal of Botanical Medicine* 1, no. 4 (1996): 2–7.
30. Damanik, R., M. L. Wahlqvist, N. Wattanapenpaiboon, "Lactagogue Effects of Torbangun, a Bataknese Traditional Cuisine," *Asia Pacific Journal of Clinical Nutrition* 15, no. 2 (2006): 267–74.
31. Damanik, R., "Torbangun (*Coleus amboinicus* Lour): A Bataknese Traditional Cuisine Perceived as Lactagogue by Bataknese Lactating Women in Simalungun, North Sumatera, Indonesia," *Journal of Human Lactation* 25, no. 1 (2009): 64–72.
32. Wilinska, M., and E. Schleußner, "Galactogogues and Breastfeeding," *Nutrafoods* 14, no. 3 (2015): 119–25.
33. Kahkeshani, N., et al., "Standardization of a Galactogogue Herbal Mixture Based on Its Total Phenol and Flavonol Contents and Antioxidant Activity," *Research Journal of Pharmacognosy* 2, no. 1 (2015): 35–39.
34. Luo, L.-X., et al., "Study on Lactation of Parturient Women Separated from Their Infants Regulated by Regular Intake of Trotter and Papaya Soup," *Maternal and Child Health Care of China* 26, no. 33 (2011): 5144–46.
35. Luecha, P., and K. Umehara, "Thai Medicinal Plants for Promoting Lactation in Breastfeeding Women," in *Handbook of Dietary and Nutritional Aspects of Human Breast Milk*, ed. S. Zibadi, R. R. Watson, and V. R. Preedy, Human Health Handbooks, Vol. 5 (The Netherlands: Wageningen Academic Publishers, 2013), 645–54.
36. Murray, D., "Lactogenic Foods That Increase Breast Milk Supply," verywell.com, July 12, 2016.
37. Lad, V., *The Complete Book of Ayurvedic Home Remedies* (New York: Three Rivers Press, 1998).
38. Murray, "Lactogenic Foods That Increase Breast Milk Supply."
39. Koletzko and Lehner, "Beer and Breastfeeding."
    Sawadogo and Houdebine, "Identification of the Lactogenic Compound Present in Beer."
    Sawadogo, Sepehri, and Houdebine, "Evidence for Stimulating Factor of Prolactin and Growth Hormone Secretion Present in Brewery Draff."
40. Luecha and Umehara, "Thai Medicinal Plants for Promoting Lactation in Breastfeeding Women."
41. Potter, J. D., and K. Steinmetz, "Vegetables, Fruit and Phytoestrogens as Preventive Agents," *IARC Scientific Publications*, no. 139 (1996): 61–90.
42. Chang, C., "New Mothers Turn to an Old Chinese Diet," *Los Angeles Times*, January 13, 2013, latimes.com.

43. Chaudhuri, R. N., B. N. Ghosh, and B. N. Chatterjee, "Diet Intake Patterns of Non-Bengali Muslim Mothers During Pregnancy and Lactation," *Indian Journal of Public Health* 33, no. 2 (1989): 82–83.

44. Chandrasekhar, K., J. Kapoor, and S. Anishetty, "A Prospective, Randomized Double-Blind, Placebo-Controlled Study of Safety and Efficacy of a High-Concentration Full-Spectrum Extract of Ashwagandha Root In Reducing Stress and Anxiety in Adults," *Indian Journal of Psychological Medicine* 34, no. 3 (2012): 255.

45. Singh, N., et al., "*Withania somnifera* (Ashwagandha), a Rejuvenating Herbal Drug Which Enhances Survival During Stress (an Adaptogen)," *International Journal of Crude Drug Research* 20, no. 1 (1982): 29–35.

46. Mishra, L. C., B. B. Singh, and S. Dagenais, "Scientific Basis for the Therapeutic Use of *Withania somnifera* (Ashwagandha): A Review," *Alternative Medicine Review* 5, no. 4 (2000): 334–46.

47. Parvez, S., et al., "Probiotics and Their Fermented Food Products Are Beneficial for Health," *Journal of Applied Microbiology* 100, no. 6 (2006): 1171–85.

48. Ibid.

49. Bowen, A., and L. Tumback, "Alcohol and Breastfeeding," *Nursing for Women's Health* 14, no. 6 (2010): 454–61.

50. Mennella, J. A., and G. K. Beauchamp, "The Transfer of Alcohol to Human Milk: Effects on Flavor and the Infant's Behavior," *New England Journal of Medicine* 325, no. 14 (1991): 981–85.

51. Mayo, J. L., "Black Cohosh and Chasteberry: Herbs Valued by Women for Centuries," *Clinical Nutrition Insights* 6, no. 15 (1998): 22–26.

52. Hill, Chatterton, and Aldag, "Serum Prolactin in Breastfeeding: State of the Science."

53. Hale, T. W., *Medications and Mothers' Milk*, 15th ed. (Amarillo, TX: Hale Publishing, 2014).

54. Santos, I. S., A. Matijasevich, and M. R. Domingues, "Maternal Caffeine Consumption and Infant Nighttime Waking: Prospective Cohort Study," *Pediatrics* 129, no. 5 (2012): 860–68.

55. McNutt, M., "Mercury and Health," *Science* 341, no. 6153 (2013): 1430.

56. Hughner, R. S., J. K. Maher, and N. M. Childs, "Review of Food Policy and Consumer Issues of Mercury in Fish," *Journal of the American College of Nutrition* 27, no. 2 (2008): 185–94.

CHAPTER 10

1. Kauppila, A., S. Kivinen, and O. Ylikorkala, "Metoclopramide Increases Prolactin Release and Milk Secretion in Puerperium Without Stimulating the Secretion of Thyrotropin and Thyroid Hormones," *Journal of Clinical Endocrinology and Metabolism* 52, no. 3 (1981): 436–39.

2. Kauppila, A., S. Kivinen, and O. Ylikorkala, "A Dose Response Relation Between Improved Lactation and Metoclopramide," *Lancet* 317, no. 8231 (1981): 1175–77.
Gupta, A. P., and P. K. Gupta, "Metoclopramide as a Lactogogue," *Clinical Pediatrics* 24, no. 5 (1985): 269–72.

3. Kauppila, A., et al., "Metoclopramide and Breast Feeding: Transfer into Milk and the Newborn," *European Journal of Clinical Pharmacology* 25, no. 6 (1983): 819–23.

4. Lagman, R., and D. Walsh, "Dangerous Nutrition? Calcium, Vitamin D, and Shark Cartilage Nutritional Supplements and Cancer-Related Hypercalcemia," *Supportive Care in Cancer* 11, no. 4 (2003): 232–35.

Miller, E. R., et al., "Meta-Analysis: High-Dosage Vitamin E Supplementation May Increase All-Cause Mortality," *Annals of Internal Medicine* 142, no. 1 (2005): 37–46.

Bjelakovic, G., et al., "Mortality in Randomized Trials of Antioxidant Supplements for Primary and Secondary Prevention: Systematic Review and Meta-Analysis," *JAMA* 297, no. 8 (2007): 842–57.

5. Rumbold, A. R., et al., "Vitamins C and E and the Risks of Preeclampsia and Perinatal Complications," *New England Journal of Medicine* 354, no. 17 (2006): p. 1796–806.

Yusuf, S., et al., "Vitamin E Supplementation and Cardiovascular Events in High-Risk Patients. The Heart Outcomes Prevention Evaluation Study Investigators," *New England Journal of Medicine* 342, no. 3 (2000): 154–60.

Roberts, J. M., et al., "Vitamins C and E to Prevent Complications of Pregnancy-Associated Hypertension," *New England Journal of Medicine* 362, no. 14 (2010): 1282–91.

Heart Protection Study Collaborative Group, "MRC/BHF Heart Protection Study of Antioxidant Vitamin Supplementation in 20,536 High-Risk Individuals: A Randomised Placebo-Controlled Trial," *Lancet* 360, no. 9326 (2002): 23.

Vivekananthan, D. P., et al., "Use of Antioxidant Vitamins for the Prevention of Cardiovascular Disease: Meta-Analysis of Randomised Trials," *Lancet* 361, no. 9374 (2003): 2017–23.

Sesso, H. D., et al., "Vitamins E and C in the Prevention of Cardiovascular Disease in Men: The Physicians' Health Study II Randomized Controlled Trial," *JAMA* 300, no. 18 (2008): 2123–33.

Bjelakovic, G., et al., "Systematic Review: Primary and Secondary Prevention of Gastrointestinal Cancers with Antioxidant Supplements," *Alimentary Pharmacology and Therapeutics* 28, no. 6 (2008): 689–703.

Lee, I.-M., et al., "Vitamin E in the Primary Prevention of Cardiovascular Disease and Cancer: The Women's Health Study: A Randomized Controlled Trial," *JAMA* 294, no. 1 (2005): 56–65.

6. Jackson, K. D., L. D. Howie, and L. J. Akinbami, "Trends in Allergic Conditions Among Children: United States, 1997–2011," US Department of Health and Human Services *NCHS Data Brief*, no. 121 (2013).

7. Hadley, C., "Food Allergies on the Rise?" *EMBO Reports* 7, no. 11 (2006): 1080–83.

8. Ibid.

9. Ibid.

10. "Food Allergy Facts and Statistics for the U.S.," Food Allergy Research and Education, foodallergy.org, 2015.

11. Malhotra, B., and D. Deka, "Effect of Maternal Oral Hydration on Amniotic Fluid Index in Women with Pregnancy-Induced Hypertension," *Journal of Obstetrics and Gynaecology Research* 28, no. 4 (2002): 194–98.

12. Bentley, G. R., "Hydration as a Limiting Factor in Lactation," *American Journal of Human Biology* 10, no. 2 (1998): 151–61.

ACKNOWLEDGMENTS

This life is one that I never dreamed of for myself, in all the best ways possible. Being a dietitian and a lactation consultant was never part of my plan, and yet the professions found me, and here I am. Founding a nutrition and breastfeeding nonprofit and becoming the executive director is another dream I never knew existed for me, yet here it is. And this book, this labor of love, this culmination of long nights lying in bed with clinical studies stacked around me, using my daughter's Magic Markers as highlighters, is beyond any dream I could have for myself. It's all surreal; none of it feels like my life. And I am honored to be able to do this work every single day.

To all the people, too numerous to name, who have believed in me, prayed for me, had faith in me, listened to me whine, and held me when I cried: I thank you. The journey to this place would be nothing without you.

Not only does it take a village to raise a child, it takes a village to birth and breastfeed one. The village that covered me and cared for me throughout my pregnancy, birth, and breastfeeding experience includes some of the people I treasure the most. Their names and faces will always bring a smile to me. In their presence, I'm sometimes awestruck that they have not only helped usher me through the most profound and life-changing experience of my life, but that they do the same for so many women every day.

With sincerest gratitude, I thank Anjli Aurora Hinman, CNM, for holding my hand and letting me know it was OK to cry and be scared during some of the most trying times of my pregnancy. And for attending the birth of my sweet daughter, Bradley, and reminding me all the while that I had the power and the strength to bring forth a healthy life into this world. I thank Dr. Brad Bootstaylor and Margaret Strickhouser, CNM, for sitting calmly at the edge of my hospital bed at 4 AM and making me feel safe and secure at a time when nothing was certain about the next twenty-four hours. I thank you both for covering me with your warm and calm spirits, for being an advocate for me and my child and for countless other women and children. I thank Kathleen Donahoe of OhBabyFitness! for showing me all the amazing ways in which a pregnant body can move. I thank you for all the lunges, wall sits, planks, squats, and chats. I thank Danielle Drobbin, DC, for introducing me to the gift of chiropractic care and for being a fountain of support, advice, and care for my entire pregnancy and beyond. I thank Theresa Kinzley for being a mentor and friend and for always reminding me to take care of myself and slow down. Thank you for reminding this dietitian to nourish myself first so I can nourish others.

To Matthew Lore, for taking a chance on me nearly a decade ago and giving me the opportunity to write about what I love and the freedom to do it in an authentic way, I thank you. Thank you to the entire team at The Experiment. Writing books has always proven to be an exhausting endeavor but one made so worthwhile by the remarkable end product—it truly takes a village to make this magic happen!

Lastly, I thank John and Linda Simpson. You have been my guides through this world for over three decades. You have taught me love, strength, and patience. You have supported every inch of who I am even when that differed from who you are. You are the most tremendous parents and grandparents that anyone could ever ask for. Thank you for making this life possible.

INDEX

accessories, for breastfeeding, **18–23**
adrenocorticotrophic hormones (ACTH), **28, 29**
agalactorrhea, **32**
alcohol, **20, 106, 119–20**
allergies, food, **91, 127**
almonds
  Almond Butter Cookies, **216**
  Almond-Lime Shortbread, **214**
  Almond Milk, **141**
  Ayurvedic Almond Milk, **142**
  Chocolate Malt Superfood Bars, **193–94**
  Cinnamon Cardamom Blondies, **218–19**
  Classic Sugar Cookies, **219–20**
  No-Bake Peanut Butter Oat Bars, **192–93**
  Snickerdoodles, **217–18**
amenorrhea, **84**
androgens, **43–44**
anise seeds, **113**
ankyloglossia, **50**
antilactogenic foods, herbs, and
  medications, **119–22**
apricots, **113**
areola, **10**
artificial nipples, **5**
ashwagandha, **85, 117–18**
asparagus, **113**
avocados
  Avocado Ice Cream, **220–21**
  Baked Avocado Fries, **172**
  Blueberry Avocado Muffins, **155–56**
  health benefits, **114**
  Lentil Tacos, **200–201**
  New Mom Guacamole, **191**

Baby-Friendly Hospital Initiative (BFHI), **63**
barley
  Barley Milk, **138**
  Barley Sandwich Bread, **166–67**
  Barley Water, **146–47**
  Barley Water Lemonade, **147**
  Beta Rolls, **168**
  Cornbread, **169**
  Creamy Barley Risotto, **197**
  Golden Milk, **145**
  health benefits, **106**
  Oatmeal Milk-In Cookies, **212–13**
  Papaya Power Smoothie, **149**

  Peanut Butter Barley Treats, **191–93**
  Vegetable and Barley Stew, **182–83**
barley malt
  All-Oats Waffles, **157–58**
  Chocolate Malt Milk, **140**
  Chocolate Malt Superfood Bars, **193–94**
  health benefits, **106**
  Peanut Butter Barley Treats, **191–93**
  Peanut Butter Malted Cookies, **215**
basil
  Gnocchi with Moringa Pesto, **209**
  holy basil and lemon basil, **113**
beans. *See also* chickpeas
  Chia-Flecked Empanadas, **202–3**
  Green Bean Coconut Curry, **171**
  Green Papaya Salad Som Tum, **188**
  health benefits, **114–15**
  Pinto Bean Bread, **167**
  Slow-Cooked Black Bean Soup, **178–79**
  Slow-Cooked White Bean Chili, **198**
beets, **113**
beta-casein, **129**
beta-glucan, **106, 107, 115**
bilirubin, **66–67**
biotin, **103**
birth control, **48–50**
birthing methods, **54–55**
blessed thistle, **111**
blueberries
  Blueberry Avocado Muffins, **155–56**
  Moringa-Berry Smoothie, **148–49**
bottle-feeding
  after breastfeeding is well established, **6**
  before breastfeeding is well established,
    59–60
  passive nature of, **5–6**
  proper positions for, **82–83**
  reasons to supplement with, **64**
  risk of overfeeding with, **83**
bowel movements, tracking, **36–37**
bra, nursing, **21**
breads
  Agave Graham Oatmeal Bread, **165–66**
  Barley Sandwich Bread, **166–67**
  Beta Rolls, **168**
  Cornbread, **169**
  Pinto Bean Bread, **167**
breastfeeding. *See also* breast milk
  accessories for, **18–23**

basics of, **9–24**
books on, **3**
classes on, **3–4**
cultural norms, **70–71**
daily frequency, **70–71**
on demand, importance of, **7, 71**
exclusive, for six months, **76**
history of, in the United States, **70**
latching, **9–11, 59–60**
multitasking while, **7**
nonnutritive, **7**
pain during, **32**
parent-imposed schedules, **71**
positioning, **11–16**
preparing for, **3–4**
successful, predictors of, **22**
suck-swallow ratios, **5**
support for, **4, 23–24**
switching breasts, **16–17**
breast milk. *See also* milk supply
   at-home testing of, **19–20**
   digestion time, **63, 68**
   expressing, methods for, **72–76**
   milk-making hormones, **28–30**
   milk production stages, **26–28**
   quality of, dietary influences on, **129–30**
   science behind, **25–30**
breast pumps
   choosing, **73–74**
   electric, **73, 81**
   expressing milk with, **72–73**
   getting the most out of, **75–76**
   hospital-grade, **19, 73**
   how they work, **33–35**
   manual, **74**
   need for, note about, **19**
   normal output from, **34**
   starting to use, **34–35**
   using away from home, **81–82**
breasts. *See also* breast milk
   abscesses in, **41**
   breast augmentation surgery, **40**
   breast reduction surgery, **39–40**
   engorgement, **17–18, 43**
   insufficient glandular tissue in, **42–43**
   mastitis, **41–42**
   plugged ducts, **40–41, 42**
   switching, while breastfeeding, **16–17**
brewer's yeast
   about, **109**
   Power Pancakes, **159**
bromocriptine, **121–22**

Burgers, Beluga Lentil, **198–99**

caffeine, **122–23**
calcium, **102, 103**
calcium/magnesium supplements, **85**
calorie needs, **86, 92, 93**
caraway seeds, **113**
carbohydrates, **95–96**
carotenoids, **105**
carrots
   Creamy Barley Risotto, **197**
   Ginger-Glazed Carrots, **173**
   Lentil Samosas, **205–6**
   Roasted Carrot Soup, **180**
   Slow-Cooked Black Bean Soup, **178–79**
   Spicy Wilted Kale Salad, **185**
   Spring Salad with Balsamic Vinaigrette
      and Spiced Pecans, **183–84**
   Vegetable and Barley Stew, **182–83**
casein, **128**
Cashew Milk, **142–43**
cesarean sections, **54**
chasteberry, **121**
chia seeds
   All-Oats Waffles, **157–58**
   Almond Butter Cookies, **216**
   Chia-Flecked Empanadas, **202–3**
   Chocolate Malt Superfood Bars, **193–94**
   Classic Sugar Cookies, **219–20**
   Cornbread, **169**
   Ginger Chia Seed Cookies, **213–14**
   health benefits, **116**
   Lemon Oat Scones, **162–63**
   Lentil Fritters, **204**
   Moringa Muffins, **154**
   Oatmeal Milk-In Cookies, **212–13**
   Oatmeal Pancakes, **160**
   Peanut Butter Malted Cookies, **215**
   Power Pancakes, **159**
   Snickerdoodles, **217–18**
   Strawberry and Oats Smoothie, **148**
   Sweet Potato Muffins, **153**
chickpeas
   Caesar Salad with Falafel Chickpeas,
      186–87
   Cinnamon Cardamom Blondies, **218–19**
   Classic Hummus, **120**
   Creamy Barley Risotto, **197**
   Falafel Roasted Chickpeas, **195**
   health benefits, **114–15**
   Moroccan Spiced Chickpea Stew, **181–82**
   Vegetable and Barley Stew, **182–83**

Chili, Slow-Cooked White Bean, **198**
chloride, **103**
Chocolate Malt Milk, **140**
Chocolate Malt Superfood Bars, **193–94**
cholesterol, **110, 111**
choline, **103**
chromium, **100–101, 103**
Cinnamon Cardamom Blondies, **218–19**
circadian rhythms, **70**
coconut
    Green Bean Coconut Curry, **171**
    Quick Coconut Milk Yogurt, **152**
colostrum, **26–27**
condoms, **49**
cookies and bars
    Almond Butter Cookies, **216**
    Almond-Lime Shortbread, **214**
    Chocolate Malt Superfood Bars, **193–94**
    Cinnamon Cardamom Blondies, **218–19**
    Classic Sugar Cookies, **218–19**
    Ginger Chia Seed Cookies, **213–14**
    No-Bake Peanut Butter Oat Bars, **192–93**
    Oatmeal Milk-In Cookies, **212–13**
    Peanut Butter Malted Cookies, **215**
    Snickerdoodles, **217–18**
copper, **101, 103**
coriander seeds, **113**
Cornbread, **169**
cortisol, **29–30**
cow's milk, **128–29**
cradle position, **12–13**
cream, nipple, **22**
cross-cradle position, **12–13**
crying infants, **72**

Dashi Ramen Soup, **181**
desserts. *See* cookies and bars; Ice Cream
diabetes, **110**
diaper counts, **36–37, 65–66**
dill, **113**
dips
    Classic Hummus, **190**
    New Mom Guacamole, **191**

elimination diet, **129**
Empanadas, Chia-Flecked, **202–3**
engorgement, **17–18, 43**
epidural anesthetic, **54**
estradiol, **84**
exercise, **95**

Fair Labor Standards Act (FLSA), **81–82**
Falafel Roasted Chickpeas, **195**
fasting, **94–95**
fats, dietary, **96–99**
fennel
    Barley Water, **146–47**
    health benefits, **113**
fenugreek
    Barley Water, **146–47**
    Fenugreek Tea, **145**
    Green Bean Coconut Curry, **171**
    health benefits, **109–11**
    Impossibly Good Curry, **199–200**
    Vegetable and Barley Stew, **182–83**
fermented foods, **118–19**
fish, mercury in, **123–24**
flavonolignans, **110**
flaxseed oil
    Caesar Salad with Falafel Chickpeas,
        186–87
    Classic Hummus, **190**
    health benefits, **117**
    Moringa-Berry Smoothie, **148–49**
    Spring Salad with Balsamic Vinaigrette
        and Spiced Pecans, **183–84**
    Strawberry and Oats Smoothie, **148**
flaxseeds
    health benefits, **117**
    Lemon Oat Scones, **162–63**
fluoride, **103**
folate, **103**
follicle-stimulating hormones (FSH), **28**
food allergies, **91, 127–29**
food poisoning, **122**
food safety habits, **122**
food sensitivities, **128**
football hold, **13–14**
formula
    digestibility of, **63**
    digestion time, **63, 68**
    elemental, versus standard, **64**
    reasons not to use, **22–23, 63–64**
    supplementing with, **63–70**
Fritters, Lentil, **204**
fruits, **91**
fussiness, **127**

galactagogues, **105, 1231**
garlic, **113**
ginger
    Ginger Chia Seed Cookies, **213–14**

Ginger-Glazed Carrots, 173
Green Papaya Salad Som Tum, 188
Roasted Carrot Soup, 180
Teriyaki Portobello Steaks, 201–2
GI tract, 118–19
glandular tissue development, 42–43
glucose, 95–96
Gnocchi with Moringa Pesto, 209
goat's rue, 112
gowns, nursing, 21
Graham Agave Oatmeal Bread, 165–66
grains, whole, 91, 107
Granola, 151
green beans
Green Bean Coconut Curry, 171
Green Papaya Salad Som Tum, 188
green papaya
Fried Green Papaya with Smoky Cilantro
Remoulade, 175–76
Green Papaya Pad Thai, 207
Green Papaya Salad Som Tum, 188
health benefits, 112
greens
Avocado Ice Cream, 220–21
Caesar Salad with Falafel Chickpeas,
186–87
health benefits, 115
Moroccan Spiced Chickpea Stew, 181–82
Spicy Wilted Kale Salad, 185
Spinach and Sweet Potato Curry with
Caramelized Onions, 174–75
Spring Salad with Balsamic Vinaigrette
and Spiced Pecans, 183–84
growth spurts, 79–80
Guacamole, New Mom, 191

hand expression, 74–75
hemp oil
Caesar Salad with Falafel Chickpeas,
186–87
Classic Hummus, 190
Moringa-Berry Smoothie, 148–49
Sesame Milk, 138–39
Strawberry and Oats Smoothie, 148
hemp seeds
Agave Graham Oatmeal Bread, 165–66
Caesar Salad with Falafel Chickpeas,
186–87
Chocolate Malt Milk, 140
Chocolate Malt Superfood Bars, 193–94
Cornbread, 169

Granola, 151
health benefits, 117
Hemp Milk, 139–40
Hemp Seed Oatmeal, 156
Oatmeal Milk-In Cookies, 212–13
Oatmeal Pancakes, 160
holy basil, 113
hormonal birth control, 48–50
hormones, milk-making, 28–30
Hummus, Classic, 190
hunger cues, 17, 72
hydration, 132
hyperbilirubinemia, 66–67
hyperthyroidism, 45–46
hypoprolactinemia, 46–47
hypothyroidism, 44–45

Ice Cream, Avocado, 220–21
infants
anatomical abnormalities, 50–54
crying, 72
food allergies in, 127–29
fussiness in, 127
growth spurts, 79–80
hunger cues, 17, 72
introducing solid foods to, 76–78
lip smacking, 17
nighttime feedings, 68–70
nighttime sleeping, 67–68
preemies, 55–56
tongue- and lip ties, 50–53
weight gain, guidelines on, 37–38
weight loss in, 65–66
infertility, 47
iodine, 101, 103
iron, 101–2, 103
IUDs, 49

jaundice, 66–67

kale
Avocado Ice Cream, 220–21
Spicy Wilted Kale Salad, 185

lactagogue, 105
lactational amenorrhea method (LAM),
48–49
lactogenesis, defined, 26
lactogenesis I, 26
lactogenesis II, 26, 28

lactogenesis III, **26**
lactogenic foods
    choosing right ones, **130**
    for family members, **130–31**
    types of, **105–19**
lactose intolerance, **129**
laid-back position, **14–15**
latching
    basics of, **9–11**
    ineffective, **59–60**
legumes. *See also* beans; lentils
    health benefits, **114–15**
    Moringa Poricha Kootu, **208**
lemon basil, **113**
lemons
    Barley Water Lemonade, **147**
    Lemon Oat Scones, **162–63**
lentils
    Beluga Lentil Burgers, **198–99**
    Lentil Fritters, **204**
    Lentil Samosas, **205–6**
    Lentil Tacos, **200–201**
letdowns, **11**
levonorgestrel IUDs, **49**
lip smacking, **17**
lip ties, **50–53**
luteinizing hormones (LH), **28, 84**

macronutrients, **95–99**
magnesium, **103**
malnutrition, **85–87**
mammaplasties, **39–40**
manganese, **103**
Massage-Stroke-Shake (MSS) method, **75–76**
mastitis, **41–42**
medications
    antilactogenic, **121–22**
    contraindicated with breastfeeding, **64**
    for treating low milk supply, **125**
melanocyte-stimulating hormones (MSH), **28**
menstruation, **84–85, 111**
menthol, **121**
mercury, in fish, **123–24**
metabolism errors, inborn, **64**
methergine, **121–22**
metoclopramide, **125**
micronutrients, **99–103**
milk (dairy), **128–29**
milks (plant-based)
    Almond Milk, **141**
    Ayurvedic Almond Milk, **142**
    Barley Milk, **138**
    Cashew Milk, **142–43**
    Chocolate Malt Milk, **140**
    Golden Milk, **145**
    Hemp Milk, **139–40**
    Oat Milk, **137**
    Pumpkin Seed Milk, **143**
    Sesame Milk, **138–39**
milk supply
    boosting, with lactogenic foods, **105–19**
    building and maintaining, **4–8**
    defined, **33**
    during engorgement, **17–18**
    evaluating, **33–35**
    foods that decrease, **119–21**
    herbs that decrease, **121**
    low, medical reasons for, **39–57, 64**
    low, medical term for, **32**
    low, nonmedical reasons for, **58–78**
    medications that decrease, **121–22**
    slumps in, reasons behind, **79–87**
milk thistle
    health benefits, **110–11**
    Milk Thistle Tea, **146**
milk transfer
    defined, **33**
    evaluating effectiveness of, **36–38**
    variations in, **35–36**
minerals, **101–3**
molybdenum, **103**
mommy tribes, **4, 23**
monounsaturated fatty acids (MUFAs), **98–99**
moringa
    Gnocchi with Moringa Pesto, **209**
    health benefits, **107–8**
    Moringa-Berry Smoothie, **148–49**
    Moringa Muffins, **154**
    Moringa Poricha Kootu, **208**
mothers
    malnutrition in, **85–87**
    overweight or obese, **56–57**
    rapid weight loss, note about, **94**
    returning to school, **81–82**
    weight gain during pregnancy, **92–93**
    weight loss after giving birth, **86**
    weight loss while breastfeeding, **93–95**
    working outside the home, **81–82**
muffins
    Blueberry Avocado Muffins, **155–56**
    Moringa Muffins, **154**
    Sweet Potato Muffins, **153**
multivitamins, **126**

mushrooms
    Dashi Ramen Soup, 181
    health benefits, 115
    Teriyaki Portobello Steaks, 201–2

neonatal jaundice, 66–67
niacin, 103
nighttime feedings, 68–70
nighttime routines, 70
nipple cream, 22
nipple shields, 61–63
nonhormonal IUDs, 49
nursing. See breastfeeding
nursing bra/tank/gown, 21
nursing pads, 19
nursing pillow, 20
nuts, 114. See also almonds; peanuts; pecans
    Cashew Milk, 142–43
    Chocolate Malt Superfood Bars, 193–94
    Gnocchi with Moringa Pesto, 209
    Sweet Potato Muffins, 153

oats
    Agave Graham Oatmeal Bread, 165–66
    All-Oats Waffles, 157–58
    Almond Butter Cookies, 216
    Beta Rolls, 168
    Blueberry Avocado Muffins, 155–56
    Cinnamon Cardamom Blondies, 218–19
    Cornbread, 169
    Golden Milk, 145
    Granola, 151
    health benefits, 106–7
    Hemp Seed Oatmeal, 156
    making oat flour from, 135
    No-Bake Peanut Butter Oat Bars, 192–93
    Oatmeal Milk-In Cookies, 212–13
    Oatmeal Pancakes, 160
    Oatmeal Scones, 161
    Oat Milk, 137
    Power Pancakes, 159
    Strawberry and Oats Smoothie, 148
obesity, 56–57
omega-3 fatty acids, 96–97, 98
omega-6 fatty acids, 97–98
Onions, Caramelized, Spinach and Sweet
    Potato Curry with, 174–75
online breastfeeding courses, 3–4
oral contraceptives, 49–50
ovulation, 84
oxytocin, 29, 61, 85

pacifiers, 5, 71–72
pancakes
    Oatmeal Pancakes, 160
    Power Pancakes, 159
pantothenic acid, 103
papaya
    Fried Green Papaya with Smoky Cilantro
      Remoulade, 175–76
    Green Papaya Pad Thai, 207
    Green Papaya Salad Som Tum, 188
    health benefits, 112
    Papaya Power Smoothie, 149
parsley, 121
pathogens, 122
peanut butter
    No-Bake Peanut Butter Oat Bars, 192–93
    Peanut Butter Barley Treats, 191–92
    Peanut Butter Malted Cookies, 215
peanuts
    Green Papaya Pad Thai, 207
    Green Papaya Salad Som Tum, 188
    No-Bake Peanut Butter Oat Bars, 192–93
    Spinach and Sweet Potato Curry with
      Caramelized Onions, 174–75
pecans
    Chocolate Malt Superfood Bars, 193–94
    Cinnamon Cardamom Blondies, 218–19
    Spicy Wilted Kale Salad, 185
    Spring Salad with Balsamic Vinaigrette
      and Spiced Pecans, 183–84
peppermint, 121
phosphorus, 103
phototherapy, 66
phytochemicals, 99, 105
phytoestrogens, 99
phytonutrients, 99, 105
pillow, nursing, 20
Pitocin, 54
pituitary disorders, 47
pituitary gland, 28
placenta, retained, 55
plant-based milks, 136–43
plugged ducts, 40–41, 42
polycystic ovary syndrome (PCOS), 43–44
polyphenols, 105
polyunsaturated fatty acids (PUFAs), 98–99
poppy seeds, 113
positioning
    basics of, 11–16
    cradle position, 12–13
    cross-cradle position, 12–13
    finding position that works, 11–12

positioning (*continued*)
    football hold, **13–14**
    laid-back position, **14–15**
    seated hold, **15–16**
    side-lying position, **16**
postpartum hypothyroidism, **44–45**
postpartum thyroiditis, **45–46**
potassium, **103**
pregnancy, and weight gain, **91–93**
prenatal vitamins, **126**
preterm births, **55–56**
probiotics
    health benefits, **118–19**
    Quick Coconut Milk Yogurt, **152**
progestogen-only injectables, **49**
prolactin
    checking levels of, **47**
    declining levels in, **84**
    deficiency, **46–47**
    function of, **28–29**
    nighttime levels of, **69**
protein, **91, 99, 117**
pseudoephedrine, **121–22**
pumpkin seeds
    Granola, **151**
    Moringa-Berry Smoothie, **148–49**
    Papaya Power Smoothie, **149**
    Pumpkin Seed Milk, **143**
pumps. *See* breast pumps

Ramen Soup, Dashi, **181**
recipes, note about, **134–35**
Reglan, **125**
resveratrol, **105**
retained placenta, **55**
riboflavin, **103**
rice, **107**
Risotto, Creamy Barley, **197**
Roasted Balsamic Tempeh, **210**
routines, versus schedules, **70–71**

sage, **121**
salads
    Caesar Salad with Falafel Chickpeas,
      186–87
    Green Papaya Salad Som Tum, **188**
    Spicy Wilted Kale Salad, **185**
    Spring Salad with Balsamic Vinaigrette
      and Spiced Pecans, **183–84**
Samosas, Lentil, **205–6**

schedules, versus routines, **70–71**
scones
    Lemon Oat Scones, **162–63**
    Oatmeal Scones, **161**
seated hold, **15–16**
seaweed
    Dashi Ramen Soup, **181**
    iodine in, **101**
seeds, **116–17**. *See also* specific seeds
selenium, **103**
Sesame Milk, **138–39**
shatavari, **85, 111**
Sheehan's syndrome, **47–48**
shields, nipple, **61–63**
side-lying position, **16**
sleep, **67–70**
smoothies
    Moringa-Berry Smoothie, **148–49**
    Papaya Power Smoothie, **149**
    Strawberry and Oats Smoothie, **148**
snacks
    Chocolate Malt Superfood Bars, **193–94**
    Falafel Roasted Chickpeas, **195**
    healthy, ideas for, **96**
    No-Bake Peanut Butter Oat Bars, **192–93**
    Peanut Butter Barley Treats, **191–92**
sodium, **103**
solid foods, introducing, **76–78**
soups and stews
    Dashi Ramen Soup, **181**
    Moroccan Spiced Chickpea Stew, **181–82**
    Roasted Carrot Soup, **180**
    Slow-Cooked Black Bean Soup, **178–79**
    Vegetable and Barley Stew, **182–83**
spinach
    Moroccan Spiced Chickpea Stew, **181–82**
    Spinach and Sweet Potato Curry with
      Caramelized Onions, **174–75**
sports bras, **21**
strawberries
    Moringa-Berry Smoothie, **148–49**
    Papaya Power Smoothie, **149**
    Strawberry and Oats Smoothie, **148**
stress
    controlling, with ashwagandha, **85, 118**
    controlling, with cortisol, **29–30**
    of new motherhood, **23–24**
sucking
    ineffective, **59–60**
    suck-swallow ratios, **5**
superfoods, **114–19**

supplemental nursing system (SNS), **6**
supplementing with formula, **63–70**
support systems
    family and friends, **23**
    importance of, **23–24**
    mommy tribes, **4, 23**
    partners, **60–61**
surgery, breast, **39–40**
sweet potatoes
    Spinach and Sweet Potato Curry with
      Caramelized Onions, **174–75**
    Sweet Potato Muffins, **153**

Tacos, Lentil, **200–201**
tank tops, nursing, **21**
tea
    Fenugreek Tea, **145**
    Milk Thistle Tea, **146**
Tempeh, Roasted Balsamic, **210**
Teriyaki Portobello Steaks, **201–2**
thiamin, **103**
thyroid hormones, **44–45, 101**
thyroid issues, **44–45**
thyroid-stimulating hormones (TSH), **28, 47**
thyroxine, **44, 45, 101**
tofu
    Green Papaya Pad Thai, **207**
    Impossibly Good Curry, **199–200**
tongue- and lip ties, **50–53**
torbangun, **111–12**
turmeric
    Golden Milk, **145**
    Green Bean Coconut Curry, **171**
    health benefits, **117**
    Lentil Samosas, **205–6**
    Moringa Poricha Kootu, **208**
    Roasted Carrot Soup, **180**

vegetables. *See also* greens; specific
    vegetables
    in healthy diet, **91**
    red and orange root, **116**
    starchy, **91**
vitamin A, **100, 102**

vitamin B6, **103**
vitamin B12, **103**
vitamin C, **100, 103**
vitamin D, **101, 103**
vitamin E, **103**
vitamin K, **103**
vitamins, **101–3, 126**

Waffles, All-Oats, **157–58**
water consumption, **132**
weight (infant)
    growth spurts, **79–80**
    guidelines on, **37–38**
    loss in, **65–66**
weight (maternal)
    excess, effect on hormones, **56–57**
    gaining, during pregnancy, **92–93**
    losing, after giving birth, **86**
    losing, while breastfeeding, **93–95**
    rapid loss in, note about, **94**
whey, **129**
whole wheat flour
    Blueberry Avocado Muffins, **155–56**
    Chia-Flecked Empanadas, **202–203**
    health benefits, **107**
    Lentil Samosas, **205–6**
    Oatmeal Milk-In Cookies, **212–13**
    Peanut Butter Malted Cookies, **215**
    Power Pancakes, **159**
The Womanly Art of Breastfeeding
    (Wiessinger, West, and Pitman), **3**
World Health Organization (WHO), **38**

yellow split peas
    Moringa Poricha Kootu, **208**
Yogurt, Quick Coconut Milk, **152**

zinc, **103**

ABOUT THE AUTHOR

ALICIA C. SIMPSON, MS, RD, IBCLC, LD, is an International Board Certified Lactation Consultant and registered dietitian specializing in maternal and pediatric nutrition. The executive director and founder of the nonprofit Pea Pod Nutrition and Lactation Support, she provides nutrition and breastfeeding education to mothers. She has written three cookbooks, including *Quick & Easy Vegan Comfort Food*, and lives in Atlanta, Georgia.